Genetics and Primary Care
An introductory guide

GENETICS AND PRIMARY CARE

An introductory guide

Imran Rafi

Senior Lecturer, Primary Care Education
St George's, University of London
and General Practitioner with a Specialist Interest in Genetics

and

John Spicer

Associate Director, GP Department, London Deanery
and General Practitioner, South London

Foreword by

Professor Michael Modell

Emeritus Professor of Primary Health Care
University College London

RADCLIFFE PUBLISHING
Oxford • New York

Radcliffe Publishing Ltd
18 Marcham Road
Abingdon
Oxon OX14 1AA
United Kingdom

www.radcliffe-oxford.com
Electronic catalogue and worldwide online ordering facility.

British Library Cataloguing in Publication Data

A catalogue record for this book is available from the British Library.

ISBN-13: 978 1 84619 207 4

Typeset by Phoenix Photosetting, Chatham, Kent
Printed and bound by TJI Digital, Padstow, Cornwall

Contents

Foreword

If you ask primary care professionals whether genetics forms an important part of their clinical work, their answer is likely to be no. This may be because 'genetics' is thought of as referring only to the care of the handful of patients with complex single-gene disorders who are registered with each family practice, and to the one or two patients who are referred each year to the local clinical geneticist. However, in giving this answer they are wrong, as Rafi and Spicer elegantly demonstrate in this highly readable introduction to genetic topics relevant to primary care.

Genetics has become part of mainstream primary care, interwoven with the daily work of many health professionals who practise in the community. Its importance has been highlighted by the various genetic initiatives of the Department of Health, and by the inclusion of a detailed genetic syllabus in the Royal College of General Practitioners curriculum for general practice. Genetics is relevant from the cradle to the grave – it is a highly significant aspect of reproductive health, and of the care of people with common diseases. The ethical issues that it raises help to clarify the moral basis of our practice of medicine.

The key objective of reproductive care is to maximise the likelihood of the birth of a healthy baby, and primary care practitioners will advise and support many couples who are involved in the genetic antenatal and newborn screening programmes. Early ultrasound examination and maternal blood tests identify many mothers for whom there is an increased risk of a Down's fetus. Antenatal screening for the recessively inherited haemoglobin disorders and, inevitably in the future, for cystic fibrosis, aims to identify carrier couples in time for the parents to be offered the option of prenatal diagnosis. The ideal place for identifying 'at-risk' couples in time to allow an informed choice to be made is in primary care, either before pregnancy or when a woman first reports her pregnancy to her midwife or family practitioner. Newborn screening will identify many congenital disorders very soon after birth, so that treatment can be offered, hopefully before irreparable damage has occurred. Families with a child with phenylketonuria, hypothyroidism, cystic fibrosis, a sickle-cell disorder or profound deafness will need primary care professionals to help to coordinate their child's care. The same applies to families with children who have chromosomal disorders that cause severe learning problems, or who have significant malformations that occur at random and unpredictably during the formation of ova or sperm, or during the development of the embryo.

When I was a family practitioner, I looked after one young man who had a sickle-cell disorder, and a family with a child who had familial dysautonomia (a rare recessively inherited condition that causes sensory and autonomic neuropathy and affects many systems of the body). The lessons that I learned from my rather intense involvement with these families influenced my practice in many areas that extended well beyond the care of these individuals with genetic diseases. I suspect that the same will apply to other primary care practitioners. The main outcomes were to increase my respect for the instinct and expertise of the patient and the parents, to lessen my respect for the 'established truths' of the medical profession, and to be even more acutely aware of the pitfalls of care by a large and disparate team.

In the western world, the main causes of adult disease in our increasingly ageing population are cancers, cardiovascular and lung disease, and diabetes. Happy survival to old age largely depends not only on our social and economic circumstances, but also on the characteristics that we have inherited from our parents. As the authors state, we cannot change our genes, but we shall be able to identify individuals who are at increased risk of premature ill health. The key role of the family history in this task is increasingly recognised, and is discussed by the authors. The challenges are how, in the context of a 10-minute consultation, to incorporate the family history into primary care, and to translate the identification of increased risk into effective advice, in order to at least delay by several years the development of chronic ailments. I suspect that the answer will lie more in low-tech methods of encouraging people to alter their lifestyle and diet, than in prescribing ever more expensive drugs. High-quality communication skills and perhaps an enduring doctor–patient relationship are essential for this task. As far as cancer is concerned, practitioners need clear guidance to help them to decide which patients to refer for DNA tests and genetic counselling. Readers will find the case-scenario approach of the chapter on cancer genetics very helpful, focusing as it does on breast, ovarian and colorectal cancer.

As genetics is part of mainstream family practice, its many ethical concerns also apply to other branches of medicine, albeit often in a less stark and frank form. These issues include maintaining confidentiality, respecting the right of women to choose whether or not to continue a pregnancy, how to balance the interests of the individual with those of the family (including coping with non-paternity), and whether to permit the sale of over-the-counter testing kits without adequate counselling. However, genetics adds two additional dimensions, namely the implication of the sharing of DNA between blood relatives from different generations, and how much regulation there should be with regard to assisted reproduction. This has led to the establishment of the Human Fertilisation and Embryology Authority. Fortunately, the UK is able to take a more objective view of families' best interests than perhaps can those parts of Europe (and elsewhere) that have been scarred by their relatively recent contact with racist and fascistic regimes. Rafi and Spicer's chapters on ethical concerns complement this even-handed approach.

I am optimistic that the benefits of genetic technology for human health will, in the future, far outweigh the dangers of readily accessible DNA profiles. But will someone looking back from the year 2030 agree? That will partly depend on whether health professionals continue to focus on the best interests of the families they care for, respecting individual autonomy and informed choice, even if this occasionally conflicts with some of the more authoritarian tendencies of the State. These clinicians will also need to be wary of succumbing to the influence of some of the present day 'isms', including the commercialism of large multinational corporations, and religious and political fundamentalism.

Michael Modell
Emeritus Professor of Primary Health Care
University College London
May 2007

Preface and acknowledgements

This book is primarily for doctors, nurses and counsellors in primary care, although other generalist health professionals may find it useful. So if you are any kind of primary care practitioner with minimal genetic knowledge, you will find this book at least of interest.

Both authors are GPs in London who have interest and expertise in genetics and ethics, and we both work as clinicians and academics. From these two contexts, we have constructed a text that offers an introductory-level description of the issues in genetics that are relevant to primary care.

We start with an overview of genetic knowledge which will be a 'refresher' course for those who have studied it before as undergraduates. We then move through the different kinds of genetic conditions that are seen in primary care, focusing particular attention on reproduction and cancer, as these areas seem to generate most of the day-to-day genetic work that a primary care clinician will encounter. Legal aspects and the larger world of genetics as it applies to society follow on, and the book concludes with a directory of useful resources and a glossary of terms.

Referencing aims to amplify the text, rather than merely being included for the sake of academic exactitude, and readers will also find suggestions for further reading.

We gratefully acknowledge the forbearance of our families, who have lost us to libraries and laptops during the preparation of this text. Their support and encouragement cannot be overestimated.

For assistance with the final text we are profoundly grateful to Caroline Starkey, Michael Modell and Shirley Hodgson, who brought their professional skills as academics, GPs and geneticists to bear with great effect. Any remaining errors are certainly not theirs, but ours alone.

We would also like to thank Gillian Nineham, Commissioning Director at Radcliffe Publishing, for her encouragement and support during the writing of this text, and not least for her skills as a text editor!

Imran Rafi
John Spicer
May 2007

About the authors

Dr Imran Rafi BSc MBBS MRCPI MRCGP MSc PhD
In 2005, Imran Rafi became one of the 10 GPs with a specialist interest in genetics funded by the Department of Health. He is currently involved in piloting a community-based service, primarily in the field of cancer genetics, as well as facilitating genetics education in primary care. He is an executive council member of the Primary Care Genetics Society.

Dr John Spicer MBBS FRCGP DFFP MA FHEA
Later in his professional life as a GP and teacher, John Spicer developed an interest in clinical ethics and law. He teaches this subject to a variety of students at St George's, University of London. He also works in the management of GP training for the London Deanery. The ethics of genetics is a more recent field of interest.

List of abbreviations

A	adenine
AABR	automated auditory brainstem response
ADPKD	autosomal dominant polycystic kidney disease
ALDH	alcohol dehydrogenase
APC	adenomatous polyposis coli
BRCA	breast cancer gene
BSHG	British Society for Human Genetics
C	cytosine
CBAVD	congenital bilateral absence of vas deferens
CF	cystic fibrosis
CFTR	CF transmembrane conductance regulator gene
CSAG	Clinical Standards Advisory Group
CT	computed tomography
CVS	chorionic villus sampling
d.	died
DNA	deoxyribonucleic acid
FAP	familial adenomatous polyposis
FISH	fluorescence *in situ* hybridisation
G	guanine
GIG	Genetic Interest Group
HCP	health care professional
HFEA	Human Fertilisation and Embryology Authority
HGC	Human Genetics Commission
HLA	human leucocyte antigen
HNPCC	hereditary non-polyposis colorectal cancer
HPLC	high-performance liquid chromatography
IHD	ischaemic heart disease
IRT	immunoreactive trypsinogen
IT	information technology
LDLR	low-density-lipoprotein receptor
MCH	mean cell haemoglobin
MRI	magnetic resonance imaging
mRNA	messenger RNA
MD	myotonic dystrophy
MODY	maturity-onset diabetes of youth
n	number
NHS	National Health Service
NICE	National Institute for Clinical Excellence
OAE	otoacoustic emissions
PCGS	Primary Care Genetics Society
PCR	polymerase chain reaction
PEGASUS	Professional Education for Genetic Assessment and Screening
PHGU	Public Health Genetics Unit

PI	protease inhibitor
PIGD	pre-implantation genetic diagnosis
QF-PCR	quantitative fluorescent polymerase chain reaction
QOF	Quality and Outcomes Framework
RCGP	Royal College of General Practitioners
RNA	ribonucleic acid
SB	stillbirth
SNP	single nucleotide polymorphism
T	thymine
TPMT	thiopurine methyl transferase
TP53	tumour protein 53
U	uracil
UKFOCSS	UK familial ovarian cancer screening study

1

Basic concepts in genetics

A historical overview

Genetic medicine covers a very wide spectrum of professional activity – from the sharing of a family history to the highly technical analysis of genomic structure. As long as there have been clinicians, there have been conversations between them and their patients about the influence of family on disease and disorder. However, only more recently has genetics emerged from the arena of research into everyday clinical care, and increasingly within the purview of primary care.

Indeed, the modern view is that almost all disease has fundamentally genetic roots, but it has taken much research and theorisation to get to that position.[1]

Most health care professionals will remember, in their training, learning about the priest Gregor Mendel[2] and his initial researches in genetics using the humble pea. They may also remember the corruption of genetic manipulation of populations under the Nazi regime, where individuals who were believed to be 'inferior' in some way were put to death, with the aim of rendering the whole *Volk* less 'weak.'[3] Clinical genetics has moved on from this abhorrent *eugenic* activity to activities where the well-being of individuals and families is the primary goal, but we do well to remember the lessons from a society where the 'weak' were not merely disvalued, but discarded.[4]

The way in which a primary care professional in the developed world interacts with genetic medicine clearly varies from place to place, but the trends are very similar. As mentioned earlier, the taking of a family history is a genetic enquiry (about which more later), but there are other everyday interactions in this field.

Basic terminology

Introduction

There is an appreciation of the growing importance of genetics in primary care and a realisation of the importance of genetic education and competency. An understanding of the basic principles of genetics will allow the primary care professional to identify genetic risk in patients and families. The risk may be that to other family members, a reproductive risk, or a personal risk. A good foundation in basic genetic knowledge leads to an appreciation of genetic conditions that could be managed in primary care and those that need to be referred to a regional genetics centre for further intervention.

Genetic-phenotype information

- The *genotype* is the genetic make-up that characterises the physical traits, contained within functioning cells.
- An *allele* is one member of the different forms of a gene that is present on a specific chromosome.
- The *phenotype*, or the physical characteristics that we possess, is determined by our genetic information, but may be modified by environmental factors.

Basic definitions and structures: DNA and chromosomes

- Deoxyribonucleic acid (DNA), which is a double-stranded helix, encodes the stored genetic information. DNA is a coiled molecule that is inserted around so-called histone proteins. This DNA protein is called chromatin. DNA forms chains of four bases called adenine (A), cytosine (C), guanine (G) and thymine (T), which are linked to 5-carbon sugars that carry phosphate groups to form a nucleotide. A codon is a triplet of nucleotides in a coding sequence that encodes a single amino acid. Amino acids are vital for protein production and are the building blocks of protein. The parts of the DNA chain that code for proteins are called genes. The non-coding part of the DNA chain leads to a non-functional protein, and variations in these regions can have important physiological effects.
- Chromosomes are thus threadlike linear strands of chromatin (i.e. DNA and histone proteins) which are present in the nucleus of cells. There are 22 human chromosomes, numbered from 1 to 22, with X and Y defined as the sex chromosomes. Each normal cell has 46 chromosomes, with two copies of chromosomes 1 to 22 and two sex chromosomes. XX is female and XY is male. Thus in a normal cell there are 46 chromosomes – this is also known as the diploid number. Gamete cells, which are involved in reproduction (i.e. sperm or eggs), have the haploid number of chromosomes. This is half the total number of chromosomes (i.e. 23 chromosomes in humans). The term 'autosome' refers to any of the 22 nuclear chromosomes. The karyotype refers to the chromosomal constitution of a cell.
- Each chromosome has a centromere. This is a specialised portion of the chromosome which is important during the process of mitosis and meiosis. It divides the DNA in a chromosome into two parts, namely the centromeric part and the free end, known as the telomeric end. The telomeric end of a chromosome is important in the replication and stability of a chromosome.
- If the arms of the chromosome are of unequal length, the short arm is called p (petite) and the long arm is called q. An acrocentric chromosome is one in which the centromere is found towards one end, so that there is a long arm and a short arm.
- A chromosome translocation is the rearrangement of part or all of the material on one chromosome to another chromosome, and it usually occurs during meiosis. This could be balanced if all of the genetic material is present, or unbalanced if genetic material has been lost or gained.
- Each egg or sperm contains 23 chromosomes, with one of each pair of chromosomes 1 to 22 and one of the two sex chromosomes. One egg and

one sperm combine to make a fetus. Each person receives half their chromosomes from their mother and half from their father. Siblings therefore share some of the same chromosomes.

- Aneuploidy refers to an abnormal number of chromosomes. An excess is termed hyperploidy (e.g. trisomy refers to the presence of an extra copy). A reduction or hypoploidy may also occur (e.g. monosomy refers to the absence of a copy of a chromosome).
- The term 'diploid' refers to the presence of two copies of each chromosome, whereas the term 'disomic' refers to the presence of two copies of a particular chromosome.
- Meiosis is the process whereby division of diploid germ cells leads to the formation of haploid gametes. The main function of meiosis is to produce variation between individuals as a basis for natural selection. All four sets of the 23 chromosomes produced during meiosis differ both from each other and from the parent cell, because chromosomal material of maternal and paternal origin is rearranged before the first cell division.
- Mitosis is the process of cell division whereby a single diploid cell divides to produce two identical diploid daughter cells.

Coding and non-coding: genes

- A gene is a DNA segment (i.e. nucleotide bases) that codes for the production of a protein and is the basic unit of inheritance or heredity. One gene usually encodes one protein. Genes are found on the chromosomes. Each kind of chromosome contains a different set of genes.
- Exons are the coding parts of the genes.
- Introns are the non-coding parts of the genes.
- Promoter regions regulate gene expression within genes, which controls when a gene will be used to make an encoding protein.
- Each cell contains two of each chromosome.
- Each cell contains two copies of all the human genes, except on the X and Y chromosome in males.
- There are thought to be around 100,000 genes.

Transcription, messenger RNA and translation

- RNA copies of the gene are made when the protein that is encoded by a gene is needed by the cell.
- This transcription process proceeds in a 5' to 3' direction along the DNA sequence.
- The 5' refers to the order in which the 5 carbon atoms of the deoxyribose molecules are numbered.
- RNA (ribonucleic acid) uses the bases A, C, G and uracil (U), which correspond to the bases A, C, G and T of DNA.
- DNA undergoes the process of transcription to form RNA.
- The RNA copy is processed to remove the introns, and is then called messenger RNA or mRNA.
- mRNA is the foundation that is used to make the protein, and allows cells to change gene expression quickly.

- A protein is a chain of amino acids. Three mRNA bases code for one amino acid.
- Translation is the process whereby mRNA is used to make the protein.

Heredity and inheritance

- A genetic disease arises due to a change in the DNA sequence of a gene. DNA in chromosomes is passed from parent to child, and thus genetic disease is also passed from parent to child.
- A change or alteration in the DNA sequence of a gene is called a mutation. There are various examples of gene mutations. A change or deletion in one of the bases of a gene can change an amino acid in the protein or can shorten the protein, affecting the function of the protein or the production of mRNA. *De-novo* mutations may arise in a fetus that were not present in the parents. Frameshift mutation, in which there is addition or deletion of a number of base pairs, may result in a transcription error. Missense mutations arise when a single-base substitution mutation results in a codon that specifies a different amino acid.
- Inherited differences between people reflect inheritance of many different polymorphisms or genetic variations in protein function.
- Examples of single-gene diseases include mutations of one gene, such as in Huntington's disease.
- In single-gene disorders, mutation of one gene copy may cause disease, and this is an example of dominant inheritance.
- Mutation in both gene copies causes a recessive pattern of inheritance, such as in cystic fibrosis.
- Multi-gene diseases are caused by a combination of mutations in several genes and the influence of environmental factors, such as in asthma and heart disease.
- 'Anticipation' is the term used when a disease appears at an earlier age or with increasing severity in successive generations.
- A person is affected if someone has a genetic disease which could be dominant or recessive.
- A *carrier* is an individual who has a gene mutation for a recessive disease in only one gene copy, or who does not have disease symptoms but may pass on the mutation to their children.

Correlation between genotype and phenotype

- Genotype refers to the genetic information that is carried by a pair of alleles that determines a particular characteristic.
- Penetrance refers to the relationship between the genotype and the phenotype.
- Huntington's disease is due to a single highly penetrant autosomal dominant gene.
- Multifactorial diseases such as hypertension and asthma reflect the lack of highly penetrant genes and possible environmental influences.
- The relationship between lifetime risk, prevalence data and genotype frequencies and penetrance enables the calculation of relative risks of genotypes.

- Polymorphisms or common genetic variants in DNA coding exist and may differ from low-penetrance mutations, depending on the prevalence.

The Human Genome Project

The mapping of the human genome was completed in 2003. The significance of this to primary care will become clear over the next decade, as our understanding of the genome and clinical genetics increases. Genetic testing, including predictive testing, will undoubtedly increase over the next decade. Disease classifications will change, depending on disease genotype–phenotype characteristics. The challenge for primary care is to communicate these advances to our patients, to deal with the ethical dilemmas that will arise, and to meet our professional and educational needs by keeping our knowledge and skills up to date.

The ethos of the Human Genome Project has been to make the new knowledge and the advances in DNA technology freely available to the scientific community. The aim is to develop new avenues in the diagnosis, prevention and treatment of diseases ranging from single-gene disorders to more multifactorial conditions, such as diabetes and heart disease.

The spin-offs from the project have been the collaboration between scientists and physicians, the development of biomedical informatics (particularly large genetic, genomic and protein databases), and the advances in computational biology. There has also been increasing sociological and public health involvement in assessing the medical and societal consequences of the project,[5] and part of the budget for the project has been set aside specifically to assess the ethical, legal and social implications.

The information that the project has generated includes genetic maps, whereby sequenced gene markers can be used to isolate candidate genes. The importance of identifying genes and altered genes in terms of disease causation, particularly in common diseases, will depend on the presence of other modifier genes as well as environmental and behavioural factors. Thus the primary care practitioner in the future, when faced with the results of genetic tests, will need to have an understanding of the concept of genetic absolute or relative risk as well as the clinical validity and utility of a genetic test.[6] New genetic disease classifications open up the possibility of genetic discrimination. The use of genetic testing that is relevant to employment and insurance will be of paramount interest to employers, insurance companies and pension funds, as well as government and legal services. The possibility of creating a genetic 'underclass' based on genetic differences, and ethnic and racial differences, needs to be considered when taking on board the new advances that are being made.

The prescribing of drugs is also likely to change over time, due to the emerging field of pharmacogenetics. Individualising of therapy based on inherited differences in drug metabolism will increase over time, and factors such as variations in the genes that are involved in drug metabolism, and new drug-receptor targets determined by molecular genetic research, will change the way in which practitioners treat diseases.

The challenge that needs to be met is the need to keep abreast of the impact of the advances that are being made in genetics. The media together with patient expectations will be two powerful drivers in the need to make primary care 'genetics literate.'

The primary care practitioner has responsibilities to the 'family' as well as to the individual patient, and challenges to the right of patient confidentiality are bound to occur when family members seek information about their own genetic risks.

Family history skills and inheritance

One of the questions most commonly asked by primary care professionals is whether there is a family history of disease. Questions are asked both at new patient registration and during ongoing management. The significance of family history of disease may not be readily apparent if the primary care professional does not recognise its importance in certain clinical conditions. It is recognised as a risk factor in multifactorial diseases such as coronary heart disease and cancers. The importance of family history has been identified by the National Institute for Clinical Excellence (NICE) in its Cancer Plan, in the identification of individuals at high risk of sudden cardiac death, and in the identification of those with renal disease such as polycystic renal disease. The Royal College of General Practitioners (RCGP) states in its genetics curriculum that the drawing of a family tree, its interpretation and a knowledge of inheritance patterns are key to the basic investigation of an individual who may be at risk of a genetic condition.

There is a major difference between how the regional genetics service might take a family history in order to determine its clinical significance, and the abbreviated way in which a family history would be taken in primary care, depending on the presentation of the *consultand* (the person seeking genetic advice about a genetic disorder).

Family history taking by a geneticist usually involves taking a history from an affected individual, taking a three-generation pedigree, making a risk assessment, developing a management strategy (which includes verifying the family history through the use of cancer registers or pathology reports from treating hospitals), and considering genetic testing as well as offering follow-up and support.[7]

Most primary care professionals cannot offer as much dedicated time as the geneticist. Family history tools are available but, like any screening method, they must have defined clinical validity and clinical utility. Most primary care practices would use the new patient registration process to elicit details about the family. Patients may present with concerns about their family history (e.g. cancer) or their reproductive risk (e.g. Down's syndrome or haemoglobinopathies). Although in clinical genetics there are pedigree-drawing programs available, which use standard pedigree symbols,[8] these programs are little used in primary care, and the problem of how to store the information from family history questionnaire templates or from computer pedigree drawing programmes on the electronic health record has not yet been resolved.

Clearly the questions that need to be asked during family history taking depend on the suspected clinical condition, and Box 1.1 lists some of the basic questions that could be asked during the evaluation of a patient who is concerned about their family history. The importance of the information that is obtained will depend on the primary care professional's knowledge of the inheritance patterns and the importance of heritability in the risk of developing a disease. The role of the regional genetics centre must be to help to formulate referral guidelines that are easily accessible to primary care and which will aid risk stratification.

Box 1.1: Taking a family history: hints and tips[9]

Pre-printed pedigree sheets are available from regional genetics centres, and standard pedigree symbols are used as defined by the Pedigree Standardisation Task Force.[7] The following information indicates the standard abbreviated family history questions (adapted from the Pedigree Standardization Task Force recommendations for standardized human pedigree nomenclature[8]) that might be asked in primary care, together with the standard pedigree symbols.

1 Ensure that the pedigree is named and dated.
2 When drawing the pedigree, the male partner should be on the left.

The proband or the index case is the affected individual for whom the family history is ascertained. The proband should be labelled with the letter P. The consultand is the person seeking advice who may not be affected.

3 Siblings are in birth order, with the firstborn on the left.
4 The names of relatives should be recorded.
5 Dates of birth of relatives should be recorded
6 Ask about dates of diagnoses, including age when affected, place where diagnosed, age at death and cause of death.
7 Disease symbols should be used in the key to follow disease patterns through generations.
8 Ask about stillbirths and miscarriages.
9 Ask about consanguinity.
10 Ask about ethnicity.

The results of clinical investigations, including genetic testing, should be included.

Inheritance patterns

This chapter will consider the classical single-gene Mendelian inheritance patterns, which are autosomal dominant or autosomal recessive if the alteration on the gene is on one of the 22 autosomes. Up to 30% of birth defects could be caused by conditions that follow Mendelian inheritance patterns, such as autosomal dominant, and autosomal recessive conditions. If there is an alteration on the X chromosome, this could be either X-linked dominant or X-linked recessive.

Other modes of inheritance include the non-classical methods of inheritance, such as mitochondrial inheritance and chromosomal disorders (e.g Down's syndrome), and genomic imprinting where the phenotype is due to the parental origin of the causative allele. Multifactorial disorders will be discussed in Chapter 4.

Classical Mendelian inheritance

Autosomal dominant conditions

- Both males and females can transmit the altered gene.
- Both sexes can be affected.
- Offspring have a 50% risk of inheriting the altered gene.
- Affected individuals have an affected parent.
- The condition may only become manifest after the reproductive stage of life has begun.

Factors that affect the inheritance pattern

Anticipation
Here the severity of the disease may worsen in successive generations. Nucleotide repeats, particularly in triplet repeat sequences, are one reason why this may occur, and examples of conditions where this may occur include Huntington's chorea and myotonic dystrophy.

Expressivity
Here the severity of the disorder may vary despite inheritance of the same altered genes both between family members and between families.

Penetrance
This is the presence of disease caused by the altered gene represented as a probability or percentage. This may occur with later age or may not occur at all. Thus complete penetrance indicates that if the altered gene is present (carried as a heterozygote), the individual is affected by the disease. Incomplete penetrance indicates that not all individuals who carry the altered gene may be affected. The reasons why this may occur include gene–environment interactions.

Mosaicism
This is the presence of two or more genetically different cell lines originating from a single zygote. The mosaicism may be either germ-line or somatic.

Examples of autosomal dominant conditions

Achondroplasia
Familial hypercholesterolaemia
Huntington's chorea
Osetogenesis imperfecta
Polycystic renal disease

Autosomal recessive conditions

- There is seldom a family history except in consanguineous marriages.
- There need to be two copies of an altered gene (i.e. homozygosity) to cause disease.
- There is male-to-female and female-to-male transmission.

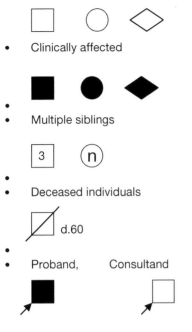

- Male,   Female, unknown sex

- Clinically affected

-
- Multiple siblings

    3   (n)

-
- Deceased individuals

      d.60

-
- Proband,   Consultand

Figure 1.1: Example of an autosomal dominant family where an affected parent transmits to 50% of his children.

- If the parents are carriers for the altered gene:
    - there is a 25% (1 in 4) chance of a child being homozygous affected
    - there is a 50% (1 in 2) chance of a child being heterozygous unaffected
    - there is a 25% (1 in 4) chance of a child being homozygous unaffected.
- Siblings of an affected individual have a two-thirds risk of being a carrier.
- Siblings have a 50% (1 in 2) chance of being affected if one of their parents is homozygous and the other is a carrier for the same autosomal recessive gene.

Factors that affect inheritance

Consanguinity
Rare recessive disorders can be more common in offspring of consanguineous parents.

Heterogeneity
If there are multiple genes that cause the autosomal recessive disorder, homozygosity for altered genes at different loci can still give rise to unaffected offspring.

Examples of autosomal recessive conditions

Cystic fibrosis
Haemochromatosis
Thalassaemia

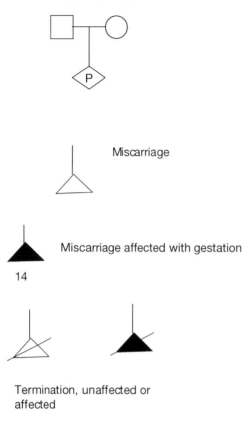

Ongoing pregnancy (sex of fetus unknown)

Miscarriage

Miscarriage affected with gestation

14

Termination, unaffected or
affected

SB29

Stillbirth with gestation

Figure 1.2: Family tree showing an autosomal recessive condition. If both parents are carriers, there is a 25% chance of a child being affected in any pregnancy.

X-linked dominant inheritance

- These disorders are caused by alterations on the X chromosome.
- The pedigree shows no male-to-male transmission, but males who are carrying the mutation are severely affected. Often there are miscarriages or neonatal deaths of affected male pregnancies.
- If a male is affected, all of his daughters will inherit the mutation. None of the sons of an affected male will be affected.
- If the female is a heterozygote carrier, and is affected, and has children with a normal male, there are four possible outcomes, namely an affected boy, a normal boy, an affected girl or a normal girl.
- The degree to which a female carrying the abnormal X chromosome may be affected depends on the activity of the X chromosome, with inactivation possible through embryonic development.

Examples of X-linked dominant inheritance conditions

Vitamin D-resistant rickets (X-linked hypophosphatasia)
Rett syndrome
Retinitis pigmentosa

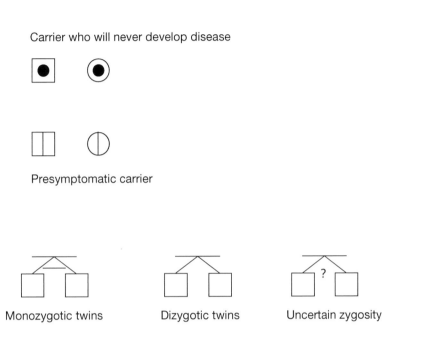

Figure 1.3: X-linked dominant family, which is associated with miscarriages, particularly in affected males.

X-linked recessive inheritance

In these conditions, the male who is hemizygous is likely to be affected, whereas females are not generally affected because they carry two copies of the X chromosome. In females, a normal X chromosome and an abnormal mutated X chromosome could be present. If there is inactivation of the normal X chromosome through embryonic development, these females may be affected.

If a male is affected, then with a normal female there is the possibility of either a normal boy or a carrier girl. If there is a normal male with a carrier female, the possibilities are an affected boy, a normal boy, a normal girl or an affected girl. There is no male-to-male transmission.

Females may be affected if they are carriers and suffer from Turner's syndrome (XO), or if there is a mutation on an X chromosome (e.g. due to a chromosomal translocation), or if there is inactivation of an X chromosome.

Examples of X-linked recessive conditions

Duchene and Becker types of muscular dystrophy
Haemophilia A
Fragile X syndrome

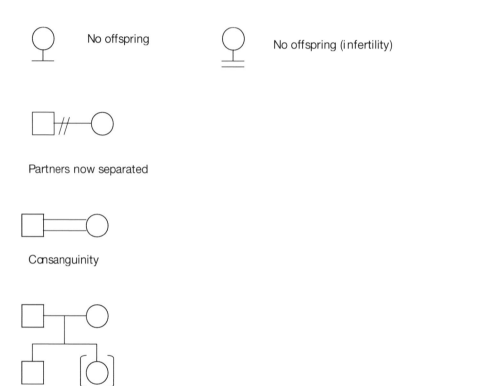

No offspring

No offspring (infertility)

Partners now separated

Consanguinity

Adopted child

Figure 1.4: X-linked recessive inheritance, where for a carrier female there is a 50% chance of the sons being affected, and 50% of the daughters will be carriers.

Genetics and ethics: a bird's-eye view

We have defined some of the central biological issues surrounding modern genetic medicine. It is pertinent to pause here and briefly introduce the ethical complications that they generate for primary care practitioners. Genetic medicine involves direct biological linkages between one person and another. Thus facts identified about one individual may have an immediate bearing on another. For example, simply finding out a blood group or sickle status, while conferring health implications on the individual concerned, also has implications for other family members. How might that information be shared with other relatives, and should it be shared at all? Might the relatives have a right to know about genetic disease in the family?

Primary care deals in, among other things, the long-term relationships between its practitioners and its patients. Usually the members of a family are looked after by the same doctor or health care team, so there will be duties of care not just to primary genetic patients, but also to others in the family. This can complicate the questions that have just been articulated.

In fact, mere acquisition of a family history and its retention in a clinical record constitutes holding information about another person without their implied or indeed explicit consent.

Genetic information that is held in primary care may also be of interest to third parties other than the family. For example, a personal or family history of disease may be sought by insurance companies considering indemnifying patients for illness or life cover. What rules may govern the transfer of this type of information?

The ethics of genetics and the ethics of reproduction overlap because decisions have to be made by patients about inherited disease, in terms of modifying or indeed eliminating the illness process. For example, couples with a family history of the serious multisystem disease of cystic fibrosis may be able to identify an affected fetus prenatally, and then decide to terminate the pregnancy. Inevitably, this kind of decision involves consideration of the value of a fetus, its value as an affected fetus, the morality of its termination, and many other such issues. Aside from the particular case, wider issues of respect for disabled people as sufferers of genetic disease need to be considered. Some may go so far as to challenge the notion of 'disease' at all in the context of inherited 'difference.'

Then there are the professional issues to consider in relation to skills and competencies. For example, doctors in the UK practise within the professional framework that has been laid down by the General Medical Council.[10] This includes a duty to maintain knowledge and skills in the relevant specialty, which in the present case is general medical practice. Other countries and disciplines have similar professional frameworks. What is the scope of this duty in relation to genetic care, as a relatively new subject, and how should it be maintained?

Genetic epidemiology and primary care

Primary care is well placed to assist in large-scale genetic epidemiology projects that will look at the effect of the relationship between genes and environmental factors on disease phenotypes, and disease progression. An example of this is the UK Biobank project, but elsewhere across the world large-scale genetic epidemiology projects are being set up.[11] Examples include the deCODE database in Iceland, which will aim to map the genes of the population of Iceland and then use this information to investigate predetermined diseases. The Estonian Genome Project is proposing to recruit one million volunteers through primary care to produce a genomic database. The Kadoorie project in China aims to recruit 500,000 people in order to assess disease gene– environment interactions.

In the UK, the Biobank project will be monitored by the coordinating centre in Manchester, with six regional collaborating centres in Scotland, Wales and

England. It is being funded by the Medical Research Council, the Wellcome Trust, the Department of Health and the Scottish Executive. This is a longitudinal cohort study which will aim to recruit 500,000 people between the ages of 40 and 69 years. Information on the lifestyle and environment of these volunteers will be collected for many years. This information will be matched to the volunteers' medical records, and blood samples will be used for genetic studies. General practitioners will be approached to collate information about patients from their medical records. Data that will be collected will include biochemical and physiological markers, and samples that will be collected will include DNA, plasma and urine samples, Read-coded data, prescribing data, and morbidity and pathology data. Encryption and transmission of data would occur via NHSnet to the UK Biobank database.

If primary care is going to assist in projects such as Biobank, information technology issues will need to be considered. Good-quality data are essential for meaningful conclusions to be drawn from such cohort studies.[12] Robust electronic records and GP computer systems will be vitally important. The current UK information technology (IT) strategy of *Connecting for Health*, (www.connecting_for_health.nhs.uk) with one unified electronic patient record, may greatly assist genetic epidemiology projects in the future. Issues around confidentiality in accessing records for research purposes would need to be transparent and be compliant with the UK Data Protection Act 1998.

The advantage to primary care of being involved in such genetic epidemiology projects is the contribution to the understanding of the relationship between genes and the environment in common multifactorial conditions, including diabetes and coronary heart disease. Projects such as the Biobank are large scale, but historically twin studies and adoption studies have also been informative. Families with large pedigrees have been the main focus in helping to determine causative genes. Genetic linkage refers to the phenomenon whereby genes at separate loci that are close together on the same chromosome tend to travel together from parents to offspring.

The spin-offs we are likely to gain from genetic epidemiology studies include new taxonomies of pathophysiology and disease,[1] an understanding of the genetic contribution to common diseases, and the possibility of increased genetic testing, including pharmacogenetics.

Risk awareness and communication

What is described as 'genetic counselling' is usually perceived as a kind of conversation between clinician and patient, perhaps with their family also present, about the risks of a genetic disorder occurring and the techniques that might be used to avoid this. It often takes place in the aftermath of a disorder coming to light, to prevent its recurrence. However, that slightly superficial description hides much useful detail and other shades of meaning that are worth considering in more depth.[13] We should distinguish two aspects, among many others, of the process of genetic counselling at this stage. First, there is the transfer of clear information about the genetic disease and the risks of occurrence, or recurrence, in the index patient or family, and secondly we need to consider the manner in which that information is communicated.

Taking the second aspect first, it could be said that competent and sensitive communication should be achievable in primary care. Those skills have for many years been the backdrop and architecture of training both in general practice and of allied health professionals in primary care. To this should be added the long-term relationships with patients, characteristic of the discipline, and the familiarity with patients and families in their own milieux. At least in the medical arena, bodies of theory and practice are immediately accessible for honing and perfecting the communication skills necessary to genetic (and other) counselling.

Communication of information about diagnosis and risk to patients is a different task. At its simplest, general understanding of complex risk evaluations is patchy at best, and the clinician may need to use a variety of techniques to aid the process. Consider the following case:

> Patient A was discussing the results of her antenatal blood tests with her general practitioner. They were all as expected and reassuringly normal, except that her sickle status was recorded as 'sickle-cell trait.' Her partner was a known carrier. Patient A had no particular knowledge of this disorder, and seemed to have difficulty understanding language such as '1 in 4 risk' when her doctor was trying to describe the risks to her fetus. He considered other ways of presenting her with these facts.

Readers will know that when both mother and father are sickle-trait positive, 1 in every 4 progeny will be affected by sickle-cell disease – ostensibly a fairly simple mathematical construction. However, even this can cause difficulties for some patients, which can be aggravated by anxiety engendered by the news of the diagnosis at a vulnerable time.

Principles of genetic testing

One of the major roles that primary care professionals will need to take on is identifying significant family histories, and referring these individuals or families to the specialist genetics centre for consideration of genetic testing. Within the centre is a multidisciplinary group of professionals, including geneticists and counsellors, who are involved in diagnosis management and genetic testing, together with the laboratory support. However, the primary care professional does need to have an understanding of what a genetic test is and the methods involved, as only then will they appreciate the ethical, social and legal implications associated with the new advances that are being made in our understanding of genetics.

A genetic test can be defined as the analysis of human DNA, RNA, chromosomes, proteins and certain metabolites in order to detect heritable disease-related genotypes, mutations, phenotypes or karyotypes for clinical purposes.[14] Thus a genetic test is used to make a diagnosis and gain an understanding of future health risks.[15]

Genetic testing may be done in a pre-symptomatic setting (e.g. in the diagnosis of late-onset disorders such as breast cancer and Huntington's disease), it may occur through screening programmes, as in the neonatal and antenatal setting (e.g. cystic fibrosis, sickle-cell anaemia) or it may occur in the symptomatic stage (e.g. Duchenne muscular dystrophy).

The aim of genetic testing will obviously vary depending on the clinical scenario. It may be to make a diagnosis, to identify carriers or to make decisions regarding reproductive risk.

The type of test is tailored to the clinical condition that is being studied. It may range from haematologically based tests (e.g. haemoglobin electrophoresis in the study of the haemoglobinopathies), to muscle biopsies (e.g. in the study of Duchenne muscular dystrophy) to DNA-based tests which assess the molecular genetics of the condition under study. In the UK, the UK Genetic Testing Network lists the laboratory tests that are available for single-gene disorders.[16] Primary care professionals increasingly arrange ultrasound screening for Down's risk assessment, and a high-risk patient may undergo amniocentesis to assess fetal chromosomes. Thus the use of cytogenetic tests is particularly relevant to primary care. Methods that are used to make a rapid diagnosis include the use of fluorescent labelled DNA (e.g. fluorescence *in situ* hybridisation, FISH) and methods that utilise the polymerase chain reaction (PCR), which amplifies small amounts of DNA.

It is clear that the primary care professional should have an idea of how useful these tests are in making a genetic diagnosis. It is important to appreciate that not all mutant or altered genes necessarily lead to the development of future disease. This is where relative risks, absolute risks and lifetime risks may be used to communicate the usefulness of genetic testing in genetic counselling. Genetic tests should be considered in the same way as other tests in that the sensitivity, specificity and positive predictive value should be borne in mind. Yet a genetic test does seem to be different in that we may be using a test in an asymptomatic patient to predict future risk of disease, and this in turn may elicit a behavioural response from that individual. Pre-test counselling is especially important in predictive testing for conditions such as Huntington's disease, for which no effective treatments are available.

If a genetic test does come back positive, as in the case of some hereditary forms of breast cancer, there needs to be an appreciation of the effectiveness of future screening, surveillance or any preventive therapy that might be available.

Other equally important aspects that will be considered in the course of this book are issues relating to storage of information, confidentiality, and social implications and ethical dilemmas that may arise. Remember that invariably one is dealing not only with the individual but with possible repercussions for the entire family.

Family issues

This chapter will conclude with a brief review of some of the particular problems that primary care teams encounter in the care of patients with genetic disorders.

First, as we have already seen, genetic problems are often expected because existing family members are sufferers or carriers, and the diagnosis can be foreseen.[17] But sometimes the genetic diagnosis is unexpected, and therefore delayed. For example, cystic fibrosis as a new case usually presents with failure to thrive and recurrent chest infections. Therefore time will inevitably pass between birth and the development of symptoms that lead to suspicion of CF or other differential diagnoses. Indeed the uncertainty that is associated with unclear patterns of symptoms, before a clear diagnosis is established, is particularly hard for parents to bear.

Secondly, for some patterns of disorder there can never be a clear diagnosis, and relatives are left with the possibility of either genetic or acquired explanations for uncharacterised patterns of illness. This is particularly the case in newborn or children's syndromes of unknown origin. Parents seem to need to know that their child's illness is recognised, to help them deal with it.

Thirdly, parents will need to be aware of the possibility of serious or sudden complications of genetic disease that require urgent medical intervention. Similarly, health professionals who are charged with the primary care of such patients should be cognisant of such risks and know what care is needed when they occur. For example, in neurofibromatosis there is the possibility of malignant change.

Readers are urged to explore any of the patient- and family-focused support websites listed in Chapter 8 to help them to understand some of these aspects from a non-professional perspective.

Summary

This chapter has introduced the basic concepts of genetics. In primary care, a knowledge of basic inheritance patterns is important when engaging with patients in order to determine whether there is a risk of a genetic disorder.

References

1. Lindee S. *Moments of Truth in Genetic Medicine.* Baltimore, MD: Johns Hopkins University Press; 2005. Here the author documents the important points in the development of genetic medicine, using specific clinical examples, and analyses their cultural meanings.

2. Marantz Henig R. *A Monk and Two Peas: the story of Gregor Mendel and the discovery of genetics.* London: Wiedenfeld and Nicolson; 2000. This is a good uncomplicated account, setting Mendel in the contemporaneous scientific environment.

3. Muller-Hill B. Lessons from a dark and distant past. In: Clarke A, editor. *Genetic Counselling: practice and principles.* London: Routledge; 1994.

4. Gould SJ. The smoking gun of eugenics. In: *Dinosaur in a Haystack: reflections in natural history.* London: Jonathan Cape; 1996. This is a very accessible examination of eugenics.

5. Collins FS. *Medical and Societal Consequences of the Human Genome Project. NEJM.* 1999; **341:** 28–37.

6. Holtzmann NA, Marteau TM. Will genetics revolutionize medicine? *NEJM.* 2000; **343:** 141–4.

7. Qureshi N, Modell B, Modell M. Raising the profile of genetics in primary care. *Nat Rev Genet.* 2004; **5:** 783–90.

8. Bennett RL, Steinhaus KA, Uhrich SB *et al.* Recommendations for standardized human pedigree nomenclature. Pedigree Standardization Task Force of the National Society of Genetic Counselors. *Am J Hum Genet.* 1995; **56:** 745–52.

9. Clinical Genetics Society, Clinical Governance Subcommittee; www.clingensoc.org/Docs/Standards/CGSPedigree.pdf (accessed 3 February 2007).

10. General Medical Council. *Good Medical Practice.* London: General Medical Council; 2006.

11. Smith BH *et al.* Genetic epidemiology in primary care. *Br J Gen Pract.* 2006; **56:** 214–21.

12. Sullivan FM *et al.* How could primary care meet the informatics needs of UK Biobank? A Scottish proposal. *Informatics Prim Care.* 2003; **11:** 129–35.

13. Harper PS. Genetic counselling: an introduction. In: *Practical Genetic Counselling.* Oxford: Butterworth-Heinemann; 2000. This is a good introductory review.

14. Holtzman NA, Watson MS, editors. *Promoting Safe and Effective Genetic Testing in the United States: final report of the Task Force on Genetic Testing.* Baltimore, MD: Johns Hopkins University Press; 1999.

15. Burke W. Genetic testing. *NEJM.* 2002; **347:** 1867–75.

16. www.genetictestingnetwork.org.uk/gtn (accessed 4 February 2007).

17. DIPEx, a library of patient experience (including this condition), can be found at www.dipex.org/sicklecellandthalassaemia (accessed 4 March 2007).

Further reading

• Firth HV, Hurst JA. *Oxford Desk Reference Clinical Genetics.* Oxford: Oxford University Press; 2005.

• Turnpenny P, Ellard S. *Emery's Elements of Medical Genetics.* Edinburgh: Elsevier Churchill Livingstone; 2005.

2

Raising genetic awareness

Introduction

Primary care is well placed for the identification and management of genetic disorders. However, most general practitioners in the UK do not see patients with genetic disorders regularly, and may have only limited knowledge of individual genetic disorders. Clearly an understanding of the inheritance patterns of common genetic disorders and the ability to take an accurate family history and to draw simple pedigrees[1] are important in identifying those patients who may have a genetic disorder. Primary care physicians are very involved in the follow-up of patients with chronic multi-system disease.

In ascertaining the population at risk, there is little doubt that taking a good family history is effective in identifying genetic risk. Recent research has looked at different ways of ascertaining family history, including the use of computers. The use of computer decision support software for genetic risk assessment, to help to educate and empower GPs in the field of cancer genetics, has led to the identification of positive family histories.[2]

Completion of a family history questionnaire, and being given an assessment of personal genetic risk of developing breast or colorectal cancer, for example, has been shown not to increase patient anxiety.[3,4] Once a family history has been elicited, the decision has to be made as to whether to refer or not, depending on the level of genetic risk. This is dependent on many factors, including the level of genetic knowledge within primary care.

Barriers to the routine provision of genetic services in primary care include lack of genetic knowledge, lack of detailed or updated family history, and lack of referral guidelines.

Over the next decade it is likely that, as our understanding of genetic disease advances, secondary or tertiary care will not be able to cope with demand for their services. For example, it is likely that primary care will have to take on the burden of pre-symptomatic identification of genetic disease through screening programmes in primary care. This will particularly apply as our understanding of the genotypes of multifactorial disease, such as diabetes, coronary heart disease and cancer, develops over time.

Through policy changes, it has been recognised that both genetic educational and service delivery initiatives aimed at primary care are important in raising the profile of genetics for day-to-day practice. The ascertainment of the population at risk, delivery of service and communication of genetic information between primary and secondary care are all areas that need to be addressed. This has obvious educational, training and resource implications.

This chapter will consider issues that will help to raise genetic awareness in primary care practice, namely:

- the drivers for change in the UK
- an effective primary/secondary care interface (e.g. an understanding of the role of the medical genetics department)
- an understanding of the importance of diversity when assessing for genetic conditions.

Drivers for change

The National Plan for the NHS

This document, which was published in 2000 by the Department of Health, cited the importance of advances in genetics and of the social, ethical and legal implications of developments in genetics. In particular, it cited the importance of disease prevention, and reported the UK Government's commitment to a long-term study of the effect of the relationship between genetics and the environment on cancer, heart disease and diabetes.

Addressing Genetics, Delivering Health *and the National Genetics Education Centre*

Addressing Genetics, Delivering Health[5] was a major strategic review for the Department of Health and the Wellcome Trust, concentrating on the educational need for multidisciplinary work across the NHS. It was produced by the Public Health Genetics Unit in Cambridge.

The paper recognised that genetics was important across the disciplines, and it called for a formal programme of genetics education, including a review of the genetics curricula and competency framework across disciplines.

To overcome some of the barriers perceived by health professionals, including the lack of teachers and resources in genetics, the review recommended the setting up of the National Genetics Education Centre (NGEC), which is now based in Birmingham. It has a wide remit in its role to facilitate the development and dissemination of resources across the many professional disciplines within the NHS. The National Genetic Education Centre has been involved in defining the core genetic competencies for the non-specialist, and has been working with the General Practitioners with a Special Interest (GPwSI) programme to define the necessary competencies required of a GP who wants to be a leader in primary care genetics.

Our Inheritance, Our Future[6]

This White Paper in genetics, which was published in 2003 by the Department of Health, highlighted the present and future impact of genetics, and the need to integrate genetics into mainstream services. It described the roles that it will be necessary for primary care to take on in managing genetic aspects of conditions. These included involvement in screening and testing, identifying genetic conditions, assessing genetic risk and dealing with patients' concerns and expectations.

An initiative that arose as a result of this White Paper was the funding of GPs with a Specialist Interest in Genetics in 10 primary care trusts (PCTs). These GPs work within their nominated PCT, their primary role being to act in the capacity of local leaders in genetics education within primary care.

The Department of Health has also funded service development projects, which have assessed genetic service delivery to diverse ethnic groups in primary care. In addition, there have been jointly funded Department of Health and Macmillan projects looking at genetic nurse specialists running community-based family history clinics for the assessment of genetic cancer risk.

The Royal College of General Practitioners (RCGP)

In 1998, the RCGP advocated a shared care role between the genetics specialist and the GP. The RCGP 'virtual genetics group' played an important part in the initial call for genetics to be part of the newly developed curriculum.[7] This was taken on by the National Genetics Education Centre (NGEC). The introduction of genetics as part of the new RCGP curriculum for general practice in 2007 recognised that primary care professionals have skills that are relevant to genetics, which include dealing with uncertainty, counselling skills, a wide knowledge base and the ability to coordinate services.

It also recognised that there was a need for education in key aspects of the management of genetic disorders, including the taking and interpretation of family histories, being aware of the common patterns of inheritance, and being aware of the diverse ethnic groups that may have an increased genetic risk, and their resistance to engaging with medical services. The document also highlighted the need to understand how to communicate genetic risk and the limitations of genetic testing. The implications for reproductive medicine and the ethical, social and legal aspects of genetic disease, including confidentiality, were all considered to be important.

Matching the undergraduate curriculum to the postgraduate role

The challenge for the new training GP is how to meet their educational needs, and match their knowledge to that required from the curriculum. There needs to be a transition from the undergraduate curriculum to the skills required for clinical practice.

The undergraduate curriculum is defined by the British Society of Human Genetics and the Joint Committee for Medical Genetics. The aims of the undergraduate curriculum are to identify core genetics knowledge and facilitate future professional development. Whereas the genetics undergraduate curriculum may concentrate on genetics theory, the skills needed by the practising physician include the ability to construct a family tree, to know where to get help, to be aware of the ethical, social and legal aspects of clinical genetics, and to understand the interface between primary care and the regional genetics unit.

Core competencies

Addressing Genetics, Delivering Health has made some key policy statements relating to educational genetics policy for the non-specialist. These include the fact that the core competencies are a starting point, that there should be depth and breadth of genetics within the curriculum, that a national pool of curriculum material should be shared, and the recognition of barriers to implementing educational change. Clinical competency defined by the RCGP is a combination of knowledge, skills and attitudes which, when applied, lead to a particular outcome.

The National Genetics Education Centre in the UK is working between professionals to develop a core competency framework that is relevant to each individual professional body.

In the USA, the National Coalition for Health Professional Education in Genetics (NCHPEG) has developed its own competency framework. These competencies for the non-specialist cover the appreciation of the limitations of genetic knowledge, an understanding of the psychological issues relating to the management of patients with genetic disorders, and an understanding of how and when to refer patients to the genetics specialist. The RCGP core competency framework covers similar themes.

National Service Frameworks (NSFs)

There have been National Service Frameworks produced by the Department of Health which highlight the importance of genetics in diseases.

The NSF for coronary heart disease[8] has a separate chapter on arrhythmias and sudden death, and cites the fact that most sudden deaths under the age of 30 years are due to inherited arrhythmias and cardiomyopathies. Genetics contributes to the majority of these deaths. Clearly, relatives may be at increased risk, and the importance of family history, leading to investigation of at-risk relatives, may lead to prevention of deaths. It is important that these relatives are referred as soon as possible to specialist units that have expertise in the investigation of sudden death.

The NSF for renal disease[9] mentions the importance of family history in evaluating patients for chronic renal disease. For example, it would be important to identify polycystic renal disease (*see* Chapter 4) and to prevent associated morbidity.

The National Cancer Plan[10] cites the importance of genetics in the aetiology of cancers, the relationship between genetics and environmental factors, the need for cancer clinical genetics services that would be relevant to primary care, and the need for genetic counselling, particularly before genetic testing.

The National Institute for Clinical Excellence (NICE)

The guidelines produced by NICE cover a wide range of clinical conditions, and the following list provides a brief illustration of how genetic knowledge may aid the management of these conditions.

- The NICE guidelines on antenatal care mention the need for Down's screening to be made available, with nuchal translucency ultrasound at 10–20 weeks and serum screening at 14–20 weeks.[11]
- In the management of chronic obstructive pulmonary disease (COPD),[12] patients who have been diagnosed with β-1-antitrypsin deficiency (*see*

Chapter 4) should be offered a referral to a specialist unit to discuss their clinical management. This diagnosis should be considered if there is early onset of COPD (i.e. under the age of 35 years) with a positive family history or in a non-smoker or with a minimal smoking history.

- The NICE guidelines on dementia[13] (*see* Chapter 4) mention that individuals with a genetic cause for their dementia and their unaffected relatives should be referred to a regional genetic centre. The types of dementia that could be of genetic origin include dementia associated with Huntington's disease (*see* Chapter 4), familial autosomal dominant Alzheimer's disease (*see* Chapter 4), cerebral autosomal dominant arteriopathy with subcortical infarcts, and leucoencephalopathy.
- The NICE guidelines on depression mention the importance of family history in the management of patients in primary care.[14]
- The NICE guidelines on epilepsy[15] indicate genetic counselling should be offered, preferably before pregnancy occurs, particularly if one of the partners has epilepsy and a family history of epilepsy.
- The NICE guidelines on familial breast cancer are relevant to the identification of women and their families at risk of breast cancer, and their management with the involvement of primary care. This will be discussed more fully in Chapter 5.[16]
- The NICE guidelines on fertility[17] do not specifically cover the role of pre-implantation genetic diagnosis, which will be discussed in Chapter 3.
- Women who have heavy intermenstrual bleeding[18] should be referred for genetic counselling if they have a strong family history of breast or ovarian cancer, if oopherectomy with hysterectomy is being considered (*see* Chapter 5).
- In the management of patients with hypertension, primary care professionals often ask about the presence of a positive family history.[19] The multifactorial nature of hypertension and the contribution that genetics may make will be discussed in Chapter 4.
- The NICE guidelines on diabetes specify the need to ask about family history, which may alert the health professional to new-onset type 1 diabetes[20] (*see* Chapter 4).

National Screening Programmes

There is also now a roll-out of the NHS sickle-cell and thalassaemia antenatal and newborn screening programme. Supporting this is the Professional Education for Genetic Assessment and Screening (PEGASUS, www.pegasus.nhs.uk) network, which will provide this education package for front-line professionals involved in the care of these patients, including GPs and health visitors (*see* Chapter 3).

Genetics Knowledge Parks

The six Genetics Knowledge Parks set up from central funds for five years were centres of excellence around the country involved in looking at the ethical, legal and social aspects and impact of genetics, as well as stimulating research. They were based in Cambridge, London, Oxford, the North-West, the Northern area and Wales.

The relationship between the specialist genetics unit and primary care

Communication between primary care and secondary care is important in the management of families at high genetic risk. Secondary care and regional genetics services, of which there are 12 in the UK, are under pressure due to high demand. Regional genetics units with their multidisciplinary clinical and laboratory role serve as centres of excellence in the diagnosis and management of patients with genetic disorders. Their relationship is not only with primary care but also across the disciplines.

In order to reduce the demand for these services, there is a need for low-risk families to be managed and reassured in primary care, particularly as almost half of the referrals into the centres come from that source. This applies to the management of patients with a family history of cancer, where referral guidelines may make a difference and help to educate the workforce, provided that those guidelines are effectively disseminated.

Lucassen and colleagues[21] have demonstrated that if referral guidelines are disseminated to GPs, they respond by referring more appropriate cases. Similarly, there are long-term genetic conditions which could be followed up in primary care after a genetic diagnosis has been made. These include myotonic dystrophy, neurofibromatosis type 1 (NF1) and polycystic kidney disease (PKD). Box 2.1 highlights the typical roles of a regional genetics unit, which may serve a population of 2 to 6 million patients.[22]

Box 2.1[22] The roles of a regional genetics unit

The clinical role – diagnosis, management and family support

Genetic risk assessment and counselling

Molecular and cytogenetics analysis (see Box 2.2)

The development of genetic registers

The development of clinical guidelines and liaising with multiple disciplines, including primary care

The development of protocols for the long-term management of genetic disorders

Liaising with commissioners of genetic services

It is important that patient data are linked between the regional centres and primary care. *Connecting for Health*, (www.connecting_for_health.nhs.uk) with its proposed NHS information technology 'spine', may facilitate this in the future. Educating and supporting primary care professionals in the shared role may be one way to include primary care in and encourage it to accept the management of long-term genetic conditions such as myotonic dystrophy. The use of a specialist genetics nurse working between primary care and the regional unit may also facilitate this process, and service development projects have been assessing this in terms of acceptability to both patients and general practitioners.

Box 2.2[23] Examples of indications for molecular gene testing by a genetics unit

Indication	*Gene*
Developmental	
Fragile X	FMR1
Prader–Willi syndrome	NDN, SNRPN
Renal	
Polycystic kidney disease (adult onset)	PKD1, PFD2
Malignancy	
Breast cancer	BRCA1 and BRCA2
Colorectal cancer	Microsatellite instability
Li–Fraumeni syndrome	P53
Multi-systems	
Haemochromatosis	HFE
Factor V Leiden deficiency	Protein C
Familial hypercholesterolaemia	Low-density-lipoprotein receptor (LDLR)
Neurological	
Myotonic dystrophy	Dystrophia myotonica protein kinase
Duchenne dystrophy	Dystrophin (DMD)
Huntington's disease	Huntingtin (HD)
Neurofibromatosis type 1	Neurofibromin 1 (NF1)
Prenatal	
Cystic fibrosis	Cystic fibrosis transmembrane conductance regulator

---

There are challenges in terms of whether primary care practitioners would be able to take over the care of patients with chronic genetic conditions. Clearly education in primary care, the use of guidelines and the recognition of the importance of a multidisciplinary approach to the management of patients with a genetic disorder will improve collaboration between primary and tertiary care services.

International and national: the importance of diversities

It is fairly obvious that there will be collections of genetically linked individuals within populations. At a superficial level, there are clear similarities of appearance wherever one travels, and below that skin-deep quality, similarities of genetic structure.

The authors of this book both work as primary care doctors in London, one of the most diverse cities in the world. As a result, they are exposed to patients with the illnesses of the world, and also the inherited diseases of the world. To that extent, London is a city of great genetic variety, and any clinician working there must have knowledge of that variety. Other European capital cities are similarly endowed with a rich, diverse population (although perhaps not to quite the same extent).

The implications of this are that, particularly in primary care, clinicians should know something of the biological origin of their patients and the genetic illnesses with which they may, as a result, present. Certainly, if they are to provide appropriate care for their patients in physical, psychological and social terms, they should know many other things as well (of which more below).

Box 2.3 summarises the ethnic composition of London in 2001.[24] These ethnicities were self-declared by the participants, and to an extent they reflect a shared genetic inheritance. It should be said that this does not correlate completely with health status, which depends on many other factors, but more with an ancestral geographical origin. Neither does it necessarily correlate fully with genetic pattern, as ethnic origin may be held to be as much a factor of culture as of ancestry. Nonetheless, for our purposes it will serve as a reasonable approximation.

Box 2.3 Ethnic diversity in London

White British	50%
White Irish	3%
White Other	8.5%
Asian	10% (Indian, Pakistani, Bangladeshi) (Sri Lankan, Arab, South Asian)
Black	11% (African, Caribbean)
Mixed	3%
Chinese	1%
Other	2% (Filipino, Japanese, Vietnamese)

(21.8% born outside the European Union)

Ethnic origin, along with variation in disease genes and environmental exposure, defines final health or disease status.[25] It is likely that since 2001, London has become even more diverse, and it has been suggested that one in three people currently living in London were born outside the UK. From a purely biological point of view, genetic diversity is a great strength, as animal populations that only breed among themselves do not prosper. It is debatable quite how that observation applies to human populations in an evolutionary sense.

An example of a purely genetic disease is thalassaemia, the prevalence of which by ethnic origin is summarised in Box 2.4.[26] Clinicians working in areas such as London, where those ethnicities are represented, need to be aware of the diagnostic and treatment issues. Clinicians working in the relevant geographical areas need to be similarly informed in order to care for their populations.

> **Box 2.4** Prevalence of thalassaemia trait
>
> | | |
> |---|---|
> | Indians | 3–10% |
> | Pakistanis | 4.5% |
> | Bangladeshis | 8% |
> | Cypriots | 17% |
> | Black Caribbeans | 0.5–1% |
> | White British | 0.1% |

As long ago as 1998 it was noted that there was an ethnic difference in the levels of care provided for patients with thalassaemia in the UK. British Cypriots seemed to be more engaged in genetic screening, prenatal diagnosis and selective termination of pregnancy than British Asians, and thus encountered fewer new thalassaemia major births. In part this was due to a greater awareness of the disease in Cyprus itself, where there were virtually no new patients born.

This experience suggests some useful pointers for primary care – that is, that we should be aware of ethnic differences in responses to, say, individual screening and health education. As ever, the membership of an ethnic group does not define an individual response, but is at least a potentially valuable part of the history for the clinician.

The need for the geographical history to be fully explored is illustrated by a recent review of genetic disorders in Arab populations, where consanguineous marriages have a relatively high prevalence, leading to particular genetic disease patterns.[28] Although the authors of the review recommend that, at least locally, part of the medical response to this is to integrate community genetics into primary care, a view with which we cannot disagree, those who look after Arab populations outside the Arab world clearly need to be aware of the customs of this cultural group in order to do so. In this instance, the social custom of the group had a profound influence on the genetic outcome. The high prevalence of marrying and having children with close relatives caused a higher rate of genetic birth defects. However, it should be noted that consanguineous marriages can have social advantages.

There are dangers to this approach, in that the categorisation of humans in this way is rather imprecise. If humans are roughly categorised by closeness of genomes, then those categories turn out to be Africans, Caucasians, Pacific Islanders, East Asians and Native Americans. Africans as a group show greater genetic diversity than the rest of humanity as a whole.[29]

These groups are not exactly congruent with the classification of ethnicities referred to above, and held since 2001 to be the 'correct' scheme in the UK. Because of this imprecision about ethnicity,[30] it has been proposed that the most accurate information in terms of genetic risk is to be obtained from explicit genetic data. This is unsurprising in itself, but also of considerable accuracy is information about geographical ancestry, as opposed to ethnic origin itself.

If true, this might conceivably have implications for simple history taking in primary and specialist care. If clinicians are carefully assessing genetic risk, they will need to know the exact geographical origin of the index patient and their family members – a task that is easier said than done in a city like London. Two examples illustrate this.

First, the disease systemic sclerosis is rare in Japanese people, more common in white races, commoner still in black people and most prevalent in Choctaw Native Americans. Where the disease is present, its severity follows the same pattern across these groups. Why this is so is not known, apart from the fact that some related genetic patterns have been found, including racial differences in the FBN1 (fibrillin) and non-major histocompatibility complex genes.[31] Thus in the diagnosis and management of systemic sclerosis, geographical origin can be important.

Secondly, susceptibility to cancer can be racially moderated such that lower levels of exposure to cancer-inducing chemicals can cause the disease. This relationship has been identified for the Cyp1A1 metabolic gene, which exists in several forms, each of which has a different prevalence in all racial groups, conferring differing cancer risks.[32]

Research in these areas is continuing, and as knowledge increases, these individual and group effects will become better known.

One last example offers a certain contrast.

In Iceland, where genetic variation is believed to be fairly small, information on the entire population is being put on to a genetic and medical information database, run by a private company called deCODE.[33] It is thought that by studying an ethnic group that has limited genetic variation, more can be learned about the interrelationship between environment and genes, by excluding the complication of geographical origin.

Where genetics tests have been applied in relation to race, stigmatisation can result. In the USA, at one time African–Americans were screened for sickle status before being allowed to join the Air Force. This practice was based on the exaggerated belief that sickle carrier status was associated with sickling crises in high-altitude, low-oxygen environments.[34]

To summarise the above discussion, we can observe that 'ethnicity' as a descriptor is a rather complex quality composed of biology, history, cultural orientation, language, religion and lifestyle – all of which can affect health.[35,36] Genetics in the classical description only refers to the first element, and is thus only one part of the rich diversity of humanity. It is important to the clinician, but a reminder that knowledge of all of these factors is relevant to care.

Conclusion

This chapter has given some indication of the importance of the way in which Government initiatives and professional groups are driving the momentum to ensure that the NHS, including primary care, will be prepared for the increasing demand – led by the public and the media – for accurate knowledge and management of genetic conditions. Ethnicity will become an increasingly important factor in the UK health service.

References

1. See Chapter 1 for detailed information on these skills.

2. Emery J *et al.* Computer support for interpreting family histories of breast and ovarian cancer in primary care: comparative study with simulated cases. *BMJ.* 2000; **321:** 28–32.

3. Leggatt V *et al.* The psychological impact of a cancer family history questionnaire completed in general practice. *J Med Genet.* 2000; **37:** 470–2.

4. Leggatt V *et al.* Evaluation of questionnaire on cancer family history in identifying patients at increased genetic risk in general practice. *BMJ.* 1999; **319:** 757–8.

5. Department of Health and Wellcome Trust. *Addressing Genetics, Delivering Health;* www.phgu.org.uk/resources/educ_project/addressing_genetics_full_300903.pdf (accessed 20 January 2007).

6. Department of Health. *Our Inheritance, Our Future;* www.dh.gov.uk/assetRoot/04/01/92/39/04019239.pdf (accessed 20 January 2007).

7. www.rcgp.org.uk/education/education_home/curriculum.aspx (accessed 20 December 2006).

8. Department of Health. *Coronary Heart Disease: National Service Framework for coronary heart disease – modern standards and service models.* London: Department of Health; 2000.

9. Department of Health. *National Service Framework for Renal Services – Part Two: chronic kidney disease, acute renal failure and end-of-life care.* London: Department of Health; 2005.

10. Department of Health. *The NHS Cancer Plan: a plan for investment, a plan for reform.* London: Department of Health; 2000.

11. National Institute for Clinical Excellence (NICE). *Antenatal Care: routine care for the healthy pregnant woman.* London: NICE; 2003.

12. National Institute for Clinical Excellence (NICE). *Chronic Obstructive Pulmonary Disease: management of chronic obstructive pulmonary disease in adults in primary and secondary care.* London: NICE; 2004.

13. National Institute for Clinical Excellence (NICE). *Dementia: supporting people with dementia and their carers in health and social care.* London: NICE; 2006.

14. National Institute for Clinical Excellence (NICE). *Depression: management of depression in primary and secondary care – NICE guidance.* London: NICE; 2004.

15. National Institute for Clinical Excellence (NICE). *The Epilepsies: the diagnosis and management of the epilepsies in adults and children in primary and secondary care.* London: NICE; 2004.

16. National Institute for Clinical Excellence (NICE). *Familial Breast Cancer: the classification and care of women at risk of familial breast cancer in primary, secondary and tertiary care.* London: NICE; 2006.

17. National Institute for Clinical Excellence (NICE). *Fertility: assessment and treatment for people with fertility problems.* London: NICE; 2004.

18. National Institute for Clinical Excellence (NICE). *Heavy Menstrual Bleeding: investigation and treatment.* London: NICE; 2007.

19. National Institute for Clinical Excellence (NICE). *Hypertension: management of hypertension in adults in primary care.* London: NICE; 2006.

20. National Institute for Clinical Excellence (NICE). *Type 1 Diabetes in Children, Young People and Adults.* London: NICE; 2004.

21. Lucassen A, Watson E *et al.* Guidelines for referral to a regional genetics service: GPs respond by referring more appropriate cases. *Fam Pract.* 2001; **18:** 135–40.

22. Donnai D, Elles R. Integrated regional genetic services: current and future provision. *BMJ.* 2001; **322:**1048–52.

23. Adapted from Donnai and Elles[22] and the UK Genetic Testing Network; www.ukgtn.org/gtn (accessed 12 December 2006).

24. UK National Census 2001; www.statistics.gov.uk/census2001/profiles/commentaries/ethnicity.asp (accessed 20 February 2007).

25. Collins FS. What we do and don't know about race, ethnicity, genetics and health at the dawn of the genome era. *Nat Genet.* 2004; **36 (Suppl.** No 11**):** 513–15.

26. Gill PS, Modell B. Thalassaemia in Britain: a tale of two communities. *BMJ.* 1998; **317:** 761–2.

27. Atkin K, Ahamad WIU. Genetic screening and haemoglobinopathies. *Soc Sci Med.* 2005; **46:** 445–58.

28. Al-Gazali L, Hamamy H, Al-Arrayad S. Genetic disorders in the Arab world. *BMJ.* 2006; **333:** 831–4.

29. Bonham VL, Warshauer-Baker E, Collins FS. Race and ethnicity in the genome era: the complexity of the constructs. *Am Psychol.* 2005; **60:** 9–15.

30. Bamshad M. Genetics influences on health: does race matter? *JAMA.* 2005; **294:** 937–46.

31. Reveille J. Ethnicity and race and systemic sclerosis: how it affects susceptibility, severity, antibody genetics and clinical manifestations. *Curr Rheumatol Rep.* 2003; **5:** 160–67.

32. Garte S. The role of ethnicity in cancer susceptibility gene polymorphisms: the example of *Cyp1A1. Carcinogenesis.* 1998: **19:** 1329–32.

33. deCODE is not without its critics. See www.phgu.org.uk/ecard?link ID=756 or www.phgu.org.uk/ecard?link ID=1340 for a discussion of the overall issues (accessed 3 January 2007).

34. Fost N. Ethical implications of screening asymptomatic individuals. In: Beauchamp DE, Steinbock B, editors. *New Ethics for the Public's Health.* Oxford: Oxford University Press; 1999.

35. Pearce N, Foliaki S, Sporle A *et al.* Genetics, race, ethnicity and health. *BMJ.* 2004; **328:** 1070–2.

36. Bradby H. Ethnicity: not a black and white issue. A research note. *Sociol Health Illness.* 1995; **17:** 405–17. A fine exploration of the various terms in this area.

3

Genetics and reproduction

Introduction

In this chapter we shall consider the issues that link genetics and reproduction. In a sense, all genetics is reproductive – it is the means by which we perpetuate our physical and psychological selves. However, for the purposes of primary care, there are some conditions which present themselves or can be identified primarily around the time of reproduction. After describing these conditions, we shall then move on to consider the wider legal and moral background.

Screening programmes in the UK

This section will give a brief overview of the genetic conditions that are incorporated into the UK National Screening Programme. This includes the following:

- newborn screening programmes:
  - cystic fibrosis
  - hearing
  - medium-chain acyl CoA dehydrogenase deficiency (MCADD)
  - phenylketonuria
  - sickle-cell disease
  - congenital hypothyroidism
  - Down's syndrome
- antenatal screening programmes:
  - sickle-cell disease
  - the thalassaemias.

The Newborn Screening Programme

In the UK, over half a million newborn babies are screened, with high uptake of testing.[1] Until recently, testing has always occurred for phenlyketonuria and congenital hypothyroidism, but now there is an implementation programme to include testing the newborn for cystic fibrosis and sickle-cell disease. The NHS Sickle-Cell and Thalassaemia Screening Programme has been implementing a programme that offers all newborn babies sickle-cell screening as part of the heel prick blood spot screening test.

Since 2002, the UK Newborn Screening Programme Centre has been responsible for ensuring quality assurance of the service. It consolidates and collaborates between healthcare professionals and laboratories to ensure that there is a seamless transition from the initial testing of the newborn, through to dealing with outcome measures. Clearly, it is vital to ensure that there is excellent communication between the professionals and the parents, particularly when positive results are obtained.

The screening pathway has been defined by the screening programme, and involves a pre-screening leaflet being given to the mother, preferably during the third trimester, or at least 24 hours before the heel prick. An informed choice can be made, and the parent(s) has the option of declining testing, in which case the GP will be informed in writing. If consent is obtained, the blood sample is collected and sent for laboratory analysis. There are three possible outcomes.

1 There may be a need for a repeat sample.
2 The result may be normal.
3 The result may be suspected to be abnormal, and a repeat sample will be necessary to confirm this.

If a normal result is obtained, the child's health records will be updated and the results sent to the health visitor and GP, with the parents also being informed.

In the case of a repeat sample, if the result is suspected to be abnormal, there are two possible outcomes. Either the repeat sample is normal, or it is abnormal. In the case of an abnormal result, the child health records are updated and the clinical referral process is initiated (for further information, see under the specific conditions listed below). This process will be described using cystic fibrosis as an example.

Cystic fibrosis (CF)[2]

Introduction

This is an autosomal recessive condition. The major defect is due to mutations in the CF transmembrane conductance regulator (CFTR) gene, which is on chromosome 7q31-32. Dysregulation of chloride and sodium transport leads to the production of thick secretions within the airways and ducts.

In the UK, the incidence of CF is of the order of 1 in 2,500, and across Europe the incidence ranges from 1 in 2,000 to 1 in 4,000. The condition is rare in African and Asian people.

Presentation

The diagnostic criteria for CF have been defined by Rosenstein and Cutting.[3] Cystic fibrosis may be classified in three ways. The classical form consists of obstructive lung disease, bronchiectasis, exocrine pancreatic insufficiency, or infertility in males due to congenital bilateral absence of the vas deferens (CBAVD). An increase in sweat chloride concentration is a common diagnostic finding. The non-classical form leads to chronic pulmonary disease with pancreatic exocrine disease and CBAVD. These forms present with failure to thrive and recurrent respiratory infections. In the newborn, presentation may be with meconium ileus and intestinal obstruction. The third form presents with male infertility due to CBAVD.

Genetic abnormality

There have been over 1,000 mutations identified in the CFTR gene. The commonest mutation is the ΔF508 mutation, which ultimately leads to degradation of the mutant CFTR. The ΔF508 mutation accounts for 70% of CF alleles with the next commonest mutations. There are some ethnic variations, with the W1282X mutation being more common in Ashkenazi Jews. The CF carrier rate is of the order of 1 in 23, with a recurrence risk for parents with an affected child of 1 in 4. The age of onset and progression for classical CF is variable, and may be accounted for by being either homozygous for ΔF508, compound heterozygous or homozygous for other non-functional alleles. In homozygous ΔF508, pancreatic insufficiency is a common presentation with variable pulmonary disease. Monozygotic CF twins are more concordant than are dizygotic CF twins.

Screening

Neonatal screening

Assays of immunoreactive trypsinogen (IRT) using a heel prick sample on a Guthrie card can be diagnostic. The aim of newborn screening is to identify affected babies (not carriers) by checking for a raised level of this marker in this blood spot. Screening is complicated by the fact that some newborns with a raised level of IRT and a CF mutation will be carriers, and not thought to have the disease. Unfortunately, in some cases CF cannot be ruled out, and parents may request further tests or counselling to identify the risks. Screening in this situation identifies a much lower percentage of carriers than of sickle cell disease.

The UK Newborn Screening Programme Centre has developed guidelines on communicating the results of screening to parents and dealing with the potential pitfalls when giving the results of a screening test. When giving a result which indicates that the newborn may be a carrier for cystic fibrosis, it is recognised that the health visitor has a key role among the health professionals, and that the results should be given by a specialist-screening nurse. It is recommended that the designated health visitor visits the parents, who should be provided with support material such as a copy of an information leaflet[4] on what it means to be a carrier of a cystic fibrosis gene alteration. The results will be recorded in the child health record. It is important that the parents are given support, and they may want further advice or support from their GP. When communicating the implications of a positive result, it should be made clear that only in exceptional circumstances are carriers clinically affected by cystic fibrosis, but that the altered gene could be passed down to future generations.

In adulthood, if a carrier individual has a partner who is also a carrier, there is a 1 in 4 chance of their having a child with cystic fibrosis in each pregnancy.

Screening in adulthood

It is possible to offer prenatal diagnosis with chorionic villus sampling at 11 weeks. Both parents would need to be tested. Cascade testing of family members for mutations identified in relatives can be offered, but carrier testing for children is usually deferred until the age of 16 years, when they can decide for themselves.

The principles of genetic carrier testing for CF are the same as for all genetic testing, with pre-test counselling and informed consent being key priorities.

Thus the role of primary care is to be aware of groups of individuals who are known carriers for the CF gene, who have a positive family history or who have partners who may be carriers, as well as identifying particular ethnic groups who may be at risk, such as Ashkenazi Jews.

Outcomes

Survival rates for patients affected with CF have increased greatly, and patients with the non-classical form can live up to their mid-fifties. Long-term complications include respiratory failure, diabetes, male infertility and liver disease, including cirrhosis. It is possible for women with mild to moderate disease to go through pregnancy, but they need careful follow-up throughout pregnancy under a shared specialist clinic with the involvement of obstetricians and CF physicians.

Medium-chain acyl CoA dehydrogenase deficiency (MCADD)

The UK National Screening Committee has been piloting studies on the effectiveness of screening for this condition by using the Guthrie test. The implementation of a national screening programme is likely to occur in 2008 to 2009.

This autosomal recessive condition has an incidence that can be as low as 1 in 20,000, or as high as 1 in 10,000 births. The carrier rate for this condition is around 1 in 50 of the UK population. It is a rare inborn error of metabolism, which leads to an enzyme deficiency of the medium-length acyl CoA dehydrogenase enzyme, causing a build-up of medium-chain fatty acids and associated metabolites. In normal metabolism, fatty acids are a source of energy reserve, particularly at times when the body is under metabolic stress. Fatty acids undergo β-oxidation, which leads to the loss of two carbon atoms during each cycle to produce acetyl COA, a source of energy. A block in the fatty acid oxidation process due to this enzyme deficiency can lead to an impaired response to metabolic stress (e.g. at times of fasting or when there is an increased energy requirement).

Presentation typically occurs under the age of 2 years, with lethargy and vomiting, seizures or coma. Of those who present as acutely unwell, more than half may survive with good recovery, but around 10% may suffer from neurological impairment, and a significant proportion (up to 25%) may die at first clinical presentation. This condition is associated with sudden unexpected death in infancy. A family history of the condition or a sibling with the diagnosis may alert the healthcare professional, particularly if there are no symptoms of the disease. The important management principle is to avoid fasting and to maintain a high-calorie intake, especially during periods of illness, in order to avoid hypoglycaemia.

Screening principles

Newborn screening pilots have utilised the Guthrie test to collect blood for analysis. The blood spot is tested to determine the concentrations of octanoyl-

and free carnitine, and if the test is positive, the newborn is immediately referred to a specialist metabolic unit under paediatric care, with the parents given advice to prevent fasting, and to give glucose at times of febrile illness.[5]

Newborn Hearing Screening Programme: genetic conditions

Historically, from the 1960s onward, health visitors would use a distraction test to test the hearing of infants. However, it became clear over time that cases of children born with hearing impairment were not being detected early enough, leading to speech and language delay later on in life.

In the UK, around 1,000 babies are born every year with hearing loss. In a critical review of the role of neonatal hearing screening in 1997,[6] it was stated that 400 children a year with significant hearing impairment could be missed by the health visitor distraction test, which was performed after 6 months of age. The review recommended a universal Newborn Hearing Screening Programme, which was deemed cost-effective. The two methods used to detect hearing impairment were the use of otoacoustic emissions (OAE), picking up sound emissions from the outer hair cells of the cochlea, and the automated auditory brainstem response (AABR), which tests the auditory nerve pathway.

The Newborn Hearing Screening Programme started in 2001 and recommends that, in the community, the screening should be completed by 5 weeks for all newborns. Babies born without complications are tested by OAE initially. Those that need special care require both OAE and AABR. In the OAE test, an earpiece is placed in the auditory canal, the hair cells in the cochlea are stimulated with a click stimulus, and the response is recorded. For the AABR test, a click stimulus is given through earmuffs, and external sensors are placed to pick up responses from the auditory nerve.

Genetic causes of deafness

Although the genetics of hereditary deafness are complicated, a simple method of differentiating causes based on single-gene disorders is to consider whether the hearing impairment is syndromic (which accounts for 30% of prelingual deafness) or non-syndromic (which accounts for 70%). This discussion will focus on genetics. Risk factors for newborn deafness in general include a family history of deafness, craniofacial abnormalities, exposure to ototoxic drugs, and spending more than 48 hours in a neonatal intensive-care unit.

Similarly, the clinical investigation of a newborn infant with hearing loss requires specialists with multidisciplinary input, and is beyond the remit of this book.

Syndromic hearing impairment[7] may be transmitted in an autosomal dominant, autosomal recessive or X-linked manner, or in other less common ways. Box 3.1 lists some of these syndromes.

Box 3.1 Examples of syndromic hearing impairment

Autosomal dominant
<u>Waardenburg syndrome:</u> sensorineural hearing loss, white forelock, pigment abnormalities of skin and iris.

Branchiootorenal syndrome: conductive, sensorineural or mixed hearing loss. Associated with branchial clefts, preauricular pits and renal abnormalities.

Stickler syndrome: progressive sensorineural hearing loss, cleft palate, osteoarthritis.

Neurofibromatosis type 2: unilateral or bilateral sensorineural hearing loss due to bilateral vestibular schwannomata.

Autosomal recessive

Usher syndrome: association of sensorineural hearing loss with retinitis pigmentosa. There are three types of Usher syndrome, based on degree of hearing loss and vestibular function.

Pendred syndrome: sensorineural hearing loss associated with goitre.

Jervell and Lange-Nielsen syndrome: deafness associated with prolonged QT interval.

X-linked

Alport syndrome: sensorineural hearing loss with a progressive glomerulonephritis and ophthalmic abnormalities. Can also be autosomal dominant or recessive.

Non-syndromic hearing impairment can be inherited in various ways, and a nomenclature exists for differentiating between inheritance modalities:

- autosomal dominant causative genes are designated as DFNA
- autosomal recessive causative genes are designated as DFNAB
- X-linked inheritance is designated as DFN.

There are many causes and different patterns of inheritance, but a good example of a non-syndromic cause of hereditary deafness is a mutation in the gap-junction protein connexin 26. Connexins are transmembrane-protein-forming channels that allow ionic transfer between cells. Mutations in this protein may account for 40–50% of non-syndromic recessive deafness, and may account for up to 25% of sporadic cases, with a 25% risk of recurrence.[8] Clearly, in view of the complexity of the causes of hearing loss, genetic counselling and genetic testing will need to be undertaken by an expert physician who has a specialist interest in the causes and management of these conditions. However, primary care professionals may well be faced with a newborn who cannot hear, based on screening results. The parents are bound to be anxious, and it is important for the clinician to have some understanding of the tests that are performed, the meaning of the results, and the need for further clinical investigation (e.g. CT scans) and molecular investigation (testing for known genes associated with deafness) if an abnormality is detected.

Sickle-cell disease

The term *haemoglobinopathy* refers to an abnormality in the production of haemoglobin. This may reflect a defect in the structure of haemoglobin or in its production. Inherited haemoglobin disorders account for the variation in production of two α- and β-globin chains that are necessary for normal haemoglobin. The forms of haemoglobin that are found in adulthood include:

- HbA – $\alpha_2\beta_2$: accounts for 97% of adult haemoglobin
- HbA2 – $\alpha_2\delta_2$: accounts for 0–3.5% of adult haemoglobin
- HbF – $\alpha_2\gamma_2$: accounts for 0–1% of adult haemoglobin.

Sickle-cell anaemia is caused by a structural defect in the haemoglobin molecule, whereas thalassaemia is caused by impaired production of a globin chain that is necessary for normal haemoglobin production.

In the UK, newborn babies are now screened for sickle-cell anaemia/disease and other haemoglobin variants as part of the Newborn Screening Programme. Antenatal screening for sickle-cell disease, and other haemoglobin variants is now being implemented through a roll-out programme. It is offered on a universal basis to all women in high-prevalence areas. In low-prevalence areas, it is offered as part of targeted screening based on ethnicity factors, or if requested.

The incidence of sickle-cell disease is 1 in 2,400 births in the UK, with around 250 babies being affected each year. Black Caribbean and African people tend to have the highest prevalence of the condition. It is inherited in an autosomal recessive manner, so both parents need to be carriers to have an affected child. Homozygous sickle-cell disease (HBSS) represents the most severe form of disease, and is caused by a structural abnormality of the β-globin chains. Other variants include the following:

- HBSC
- HBS β-thalassaemia
- HBSD-Punjab.

Sickle-cell disease is caused by a base change in the β-globin gene at position 6, where valine is substituted for glutamic acid. The characteristic feature of HBSS disease is the occlusion of small blood vessels, particularly at times when the body is under metabolic stress, leading to painful vaso-occlusive crises and end-organ damage. These patients are also vulnerable to infection, particularly pneumococcal septicaemia, chronic anaemia, and musculoskeletal pains with severe joint disease. Children may present with delayed growth, and other complications include splenic atrophy due to infarcts, renal papillary necrosis and renal tubular disease, and heart disease. Pregnant women affected with sickle-cell disease may develop serious complications, particularly if they are dehydrated or anaesthetised.

Affected babies should receive daily penicillin for life. They should also be immunised with antipneumococcal vaccine.

Screening[9]

The main aim of screening for sickle-cell disease during the antenatal period is to detect single carriers and carrier couples for the disease, so that couples can be informed. They then have the choice of prenatal diagnosis to allow them to consider the reproductive options. Antenatal screening includes a full discussion of prenatal diagnosis using CVS. The actual test can involve biochemical tests, such as haemoglobin electrophoresis and HPLC, or molecular DNA analysis. When screening the newborn, the objective is to allow the identification and early treatment of affected individuals and to start treatment with penicillin in order to prevent life-threatening infections.

The screening cascade[10] for antenatal and newborn screening for haemoglobin disorders has been defined, and applies equally to testing for sickle-cell disease as well as the thalassaemias (see below). For pregnant women, a full blood count and HPLC analysis is performed, usually at the booking visit by the midwife.

- If the woman is found not to be a carrier, the couple are deemed to be at low risk and the baby that is born will be incorporated within the Newborn Screening Programme.
- If the woman is found to be a carrier, the biological father needs to be tested. A dilemma clearly exists if paternity is unclear. If both partners are deemed to be carriers, this would be considered a high-risk pregnancy and prenatal diagnosis should be offered, or neonatal screening if prenatal diagnosis is declined. If the biological father is not a carrier, the pregnancy is deemed to be low risk. If the father refuses to be tested or it is not possible to contact him, the pregnancy should be treated as high risk.

Clearly, during the screening cascade, there need to be clear lines of communication between professionals, including obstetricians, midwifes, GPs, health visitors and laboratory staff. As part of the antenatal and newborn screening programme, a programme of education known as PEGASUS (Professional Education for Genetic Assessment and Screening) has been commissioned. This is based at the University of Nottingham and is aimed at front-line staff, but also includes specialist counsellors and public health staff.[11]

Thalassaemia

The prevalence of thalassaemia is lower than that of sickle-cell disease. The condition occurs if there is abnormal production of either the α- or β-globin chains. The inheritance pattern is autosomal recessive.

α-Thalassaemia is characterised by a reduction in the production of the α-globin chains. Normal chromosomes carry two α-chains, so the normal genotype would be αα/αα. Thus the severity of disease is determined by the number of functional genes. The α-thalassaemia trait has two functioning genes and is associated with a mild hypochromic microcytic anaemia (and as such it may be confused with iron-deficiency anaemia). It is more common in people from the Far East. Loss of three or more chains leads to severe disease and haemolytic anaemias. Homozygous α-thalassaemia major leads to death *in utero* in the majority of cases, as affected fetuses do not produce any β-chains.

In normal β-chain production, two β-chains are produced in total. Thus in the homozygous state, otherwise known as β-thalassaemia, there is an inability to produce β-globin chains, which results in an excess of α-globin chains and thus premature destruction in the bone marrow of red cell precursors associated with the precipitation of the α-chains.[12] Individuals with β-thalassaemia major have transfusion-dependent anaemia with associated long-term complications, including the possible need for splenectomy to treat hypersplenism. There is a risk of iron overload, leading to cardiac and liver complications.

Bone-marrow transplantation is considered for this condition in up to one-third of cases. Extramedullary erythropoiesis leads to skeletal deformities if left untreated, but not in well-managed cases. In thalassaemia carriers, there may be only a mild hypochromic microcytic anaemia. The prevalence rates of β-thalassaemia major vary depending on ethnicity, and the condition is more common in India, Africa and around the Mediterranean.

The genotype may not necessarily follow the phenotype, with β-thalassaemia intermedia reflecting a diverse group of β-thalassaemia conditions. The diversity is due to the large number of recorded mutations identified in β-globin genes, some of which lead to a slight reduction in β-globin production.

Screening

Antenatal screening for the thalassaemias occurs at the same time as that for sickle-cell disease, and the process has been described above.[8] The screening test consists of a full blood count and either HPLC or haemoglobin electrophoresis. The mean cell haemoglobin (MCH) reflects the amount of haemoglobin in each cell, and a low MCH (<27 pg) indicates small red blood cells or microcytosis. Iron deficiency may give rise to a microcytosis, and the ferritin level should be measured. For a diagnosis of α-thalassaemia to be made, DNA analysis is usually required, and in the case of β-thalassaemia there is usually elevation of HbA_2, which is measured by HPLC. Elevation of HbF is found in β-thalassaemia major.

The role of the Human Fertilisation and Embryology Authority

The way in which genetic issues or, more widely, all issues relating to assisted reproduction are regulated and controlled is a very challenging area to consider.

In the UK, as a response to the *Report of the Committee of Enquiry into Human Fertilisation and Embryology*[13] under Dame Mary Warnock, Parliament considered and passed the Human Fertilisation and Embryology Act 1990. This contained a clause which brought the Human Fertilisation and Embryology Authority (HFEA) into being. Significantly, it was the first regulatory body of this type to be created anywhere in the world, and it was charged with overall regulation of the field.

The HFEA has many functions, including licensing premises and clinics that offer *in-vitro* fertilisation and donor insemination procedures, monitoring research into these procedures, and regulating gamete storage and use. By virtue of these activities, the HFEA is clearly involved with reproductive complexities, which in one respect are automatically genetic as well. However, as is set out in its latest corporate plan, the HFEA will be addressing questions that include the following:

- whether families should be able to avoid genetic disease
- whether couples should be able to choose the gender of their children
- whether some assisted reproductive technologies can damage the welfare of children created in this way.[14]

It can be seen that the HFEA is a statutory body. Its make-up and functions are determined by Parliament, and its decisions are binding (subject to judicial review when actioned).

Other countries around the world have since created similar bodies with more or less the same roles – for example, the Infertility Treatment Authority in the State of Victoria, Australia,[15] and the Agence de la Biomédecine in France,[16] among others.

Some jurisdictions do not have regulatory authorities as such. This is most notable in the USA, where their place is taken by a patchwork of advisory bodies at state level, allied to various statutes and common law judgements.[17] Advisory and quasi-judicial bodies also exist in the UK, as an influence on the decision making of the HFEA and the Government itself. The Human Genetics Commission (HGC) and the Genetic Interest Group (GIG) are examples of these bodies, representing the opinion of interested parties, including patients and families.

In 2006, the HGC produced a report entitled *Making Babies* which, among other things, supported pre-implantation genetic diagnosis for disease testing only, rather than for gender testing.[18]

Pre-implantation genetic diagnosis (PIGD)

Case study

Consider a couple who are both carriers for the β-thalassaemia trait. They have an affected child with β-thalassaemia major. They have discussed their options with the genetic centre, and they feel that termination of pregnancy is unacceptable to them. They have heard about pre-implantation genetic diagnosis and would like to consider this. They are aware that 95% of patients can be cured by bone-marrow transplantation from siblings with an identical human leucocyte antigen (HLA) typing.[19] HLA typing allows an assessment of compatibility between donors and recipients in transplantation.

It is possible to make a diagnosis of β-thalassaemia prenatally by chorionic villus sampling. However, this is not suitable for couples who would not consider termination of pregnancy and do not want an affected fetus. Pre-implanation genetic diagnosis (PIGD) is a method that uses *in-vitro* fertilisation to produce embryos. After fertilisation these embryos are biopsied, usually at around day 3 when six or more cells are present, but sampling can be done on day 5 or 6. Unaffected embryos are then transferred and implanted. Intracytoplasmic sperm injection is used if the sperm quality is poor. Techniques used for the analysis of DNA include the fluorescence probes (fluorescence *in situ* hybridisation, FISH) and amplification of DNA (polymerase chain reaction, PCR) collected through biopsy. There is still a 5% chance of obtaining false-negative results with these techniques.

PIGD is used for couples who have had recurrent miscarriages, for infertile couples for whom a genetic disorder is the cause of their infertility, for cases where there is evidence of chromosomal aneuploidy in either partner, and for couples who are at risk of having a child with a genetic disorder such as sickle-cell disease or cystic fibrosis.[20]

The European Society for Human Reproduction and Embryology PIGD consortium gathers data from over 25 PIGD centres throughout Europe, and there are over 30 listed monogenic disorders for which PIGD has been used (*see* Box 3.2).

Box 3.2 Typical conditions for which PIGD is offered

Autosomal dominant conditions
Huntington's disease
Marfan's syndrome
Myotonic dystrophy
Autosomal recessive conditions
Cystic fibrosis
Thalassaemia
Spinal muscular atrophy
X-linked inheritance
Duchenne/Becker's muscular dystrophy
Fragile X syndrome
Haemophilia
Chromosomal conditions
Translocations
Aneuploidy

In the UK, PIGD regulation is controlled by the HFEA. They have allowed HLA typing with PIGD so that the offspring may be a donor of cord blood stem cells to treat an affected sibling. There are NHS PIGD centres in Scotland (one centre in Glasgow) and England (three centres in London). Each case that requires funding for PIGD is considered individually. Most of their referrals come from the clinical genetic centres, and the cost of one cycle of PIGD can be over £4,000. Live birth rates per couple of over 25% have been cited.[21]

The advantages of PIGD are that it is a possible treatment option for couples who would find termination of pregnancy unacceptable, it may reduce the miscarriage rate due to genetic disorder, and importantly it may prevent the birth of a child with a serious genetic disorder. Its disadvantages include low live birth rates, the technological limitations of the analysis of DNA, the psychological stress associated with the procedure, and the uncertainty about the long-term effects on the offspring.

Couples who may be considered for PIGD are clearly well counselled, and there is a role for primary care to offer support and information. There need to be strong links between the PIGD centres and primary care, so that primary care professionals are fully aware of what is being offered, what methods are used and what the potential outcomes may be, including complications of treatment.

Ethical issues in reproduction

So far, this chapter has described and defined the important aspects of genetic conditions with specific reference to reproduction. The moral implications will now be considered. Moral concerns in reproduction did not begin with Dame Mary Warnock's report (see above), but to a large extent brought them into the arena of public debate, following on from the first baby born as a result of *in-vitro* fertilisation.

Several questions are worth considering.

- Is it right to interfere with reproductive processes at all?
- Is it right to interfere with the transmission of heritable material in order to improve human function, or to reduce the impact of disease?
- Is it right to prevent the birth of genetically diseased individuals?

Clearly the answers – if there are answers – to these questions overlap, so they will be discussed together.

It could be argued that we have no business interfering with the complicated business of producing the next generation. It is simply a matter of the natural order of events, or God's will (should one accept such a view), that babies are born to some people and not others. Such a view would deny clinicians any role in assisting couples who find themselves unable to have children, and is probable inconsistent with a modern duty of care. The mechanics and resourcing of assisted conception are subjects beyond the scope of this book, although modern genetic medicine does call on techniques of assisted conception to do its work.

However, the genetic strand to the first question is larger in scope. Even if it is accepted that it is morally right to be able to assist couples with their impaired fertility, it does not automatically follow that it is right to interfere with germ-line transmission. This can work in several ways. As we have seen, gametes can be selected before fertilisation, embryos or fetuses can be selected after fertilisation and, increasingly, late fetuses can be treated *in utero.*

The rather strict view described above would proscribe any interference with the germ line of humans on religious or other grounds. It might be considered in some sense unnatural to try to adjust what happens as result of 'normal' reproductive processes. There are powerful counter-arguments to this, which to some extent any primary care clinician who is involved in genetic medicine must implicitly or explicitly espouse.

First, bringing about a state of affairs where an individual is born without a genetic disease that he or she would otherwise have suffered, as a result of a clinical intervention, can be held to be a good thing. Suffering has been avoided, and the clinician who was involved behaved in a morally correct manner.

Secondly, humans have been interfering with the genetics of non-humans for thousands of years by manipulating the breeding of domesticated farm animals and the like. Without knowledge of Mendelian genetics, our predecessors have, mainly in the cause of food production, bred strong disease-free characteristics in domesticated animals. This has been to our individual and collective advantage, and if this is so, similar advantages may accrue to genetic manipulation in humans.

Thirdly, note might be taken of the fact that couples are already engaging in a kind of genetic manipulation in the choices that they make of each other, without any access to high-technology assistance. Simply by choosing one partner over another, we are exercising a genetic choice (e.g. of appearance, ethnicity or intelligence). After our children are born, we (generally) try to make choices for them that are directed towards their long-term benefit. In these ways, we maximise and augment the genetic input to their welfare. If this is so, how can there be a difference with regard to genetic manipulation of the next generation?[22]

Thornier ethical problems surface where genetic choices about the next generation may lead to the destruction of affected individuals *in utero*.

Consider the following case:

Case study

A young woman, F, who was 12 weeks pregnant, consulted her general practitioner for antenatal care. The routine tests revealed that she had the β-thalassaemia trait. After discussion, her husband was tested and was also found to have the β-thalassaemia trait.

Eventually they agreed that F's fetus should be tested via chorionic villus sampling in the full knowledge of the possible outcomes, and it transpired that the fetus was β-thalassaemia disease homozygous positive.

F and her husband elected to terminate the pregnancy.

The moral analysis of this kind of situation is complex. At one point on the spectrum of moral attitudes is the view, similar to the unreconstructed view articulated above, that this is just plain wrong.

F's fetus has had a moral right to life taken away, and the parents and clinicians have been party to a deliberate killing of a person. It is an insult to the principle of the sanctity of life that this termination has proceeded. Furthermore, the fact that F's fetus would turn out to have a serious and untreatable disease is irrelevant – the clinicians involved would maintain a duty of care when birth occurred, and would look after the baby for as long as was needed. The stage of pregnancy at which the termination occurred was also irrelevant, as the fetus had a right to life from the moment of its conception. In other words, selective termination of pregnancy is not a morally valid tool in the treatment of genetic disease.

Even where this is the case, and parents hold to sanctity-of-life principles which proscribe termination of pregnancy for any reason, there may be quandaries for the clinician. What should a GP or specialist do in cases where the parents may wish for predictive testing, in the presence of an adverse family history of Huntington's disease, but would not terminate the pregnancy if the disease was identified in the fetus? This dilemma has been explored recently in the literature, mainly from the perspective of the doctor.[23] On one side were the arguments that supported parents' access to as much information as possible about their pregnancy, whatever the outcome or decision making. On the other were the long lag time before Huntington's disease becomes manifest (usually at around the age of 37 years), in contrast to the haemoglobinopathies, where disease is lifelong. It was observed that 'we are not provided with genetic printouts at birth ... long may it remain so.'[24] To which we might add that we are not provided with such printouts yet.

At the other end of the moral spectrum, the arguments might run rather like this. F and her husband are exercising their own autonomous choice in preventing the birth of a baby whom they elect not to bear. They look to the future, where an unaffected baby can be identified and preferred. The fetus is not a person, and thus cannot be killed in the same sense as a child can be killed, until after it is born. Doctors do not have a duty of care to a fetus, as it has no legal rights until birth. If F's fetus had been allowed to continue until birth, it would have been a 'wrongful' life.[25]

Readers will no doubt recognise their own moral positions at either end of the spectrum, or somewhere in between. Some aspects deserve a rather more detailed examination.

Some authors have recently defined a notion of 'procreative beneficence', which seeks to extend the principle of beneficence[26] (i.e. that clinicians should do their patients good) to one in which parents should always seek the best for, and in, their offspring. Specifically, they should seek the child who is likely to lead the 'best' life out of a range of children they might have.[27] By implication, children who are 'imperfect' in some way, such as those with thalassaemia, are valued less than those who are not so afflicted, and should not be caused to exist if there is an alternative. This view is in conflict with much of the recent work of pressure groups such as the UK Disabled People's Council, which finds this kind of relative valuation of individuals quite abhorrent.[28]

That said, there are distinctions to be made between different severities of congenital disorder. Termination of pregnancy due to the presence of severe genetic disease leading to severe physical or mental handicap might be held to be morally permissible, whereas termination of pregnancy for less severe disease might not be. Consider the following case:

Case study

G is 24 weeks pregnant, and at a routine antenatal scan finds that the fetus has a moderately severe cleft lip and palate. The ultrasonographer had been alerted to this possibility by G mentioning a family history of clefts. G is referred to an expert surgical specialist, who considers that the lesion visible on the scan is eminently treatable.

G has long discussions about this abnormality with her primary care team, and concludes that a termination of pregnancy at this stage would not be right, and in any event the degree of congenital disorder is not sufficient for her to wish to terminate the pregnancy, being for the most part amenable to treatment.

There are obviously degrees of disease that become evident during pregnancy, often considered in advance because of a previous family history. G considered that, in making a decision about termination, the severity of the condition was relevant. She did not automatically proscribe termination to herself, but gave it some consideration, and discussed it with her clinical advisers. She also held a view about the moral status of her fetus. For G, 24 weeks' gestation was too late for termination even in the presence of an abnormality. Perhaps she might have felt differently if the cleft had been diagnosed at an early stage of pregnancy.

Certainly we might accord moral value to different stages of fetal development, such that a termination of pregnancy is permissible at an early stage where there are few 'human' characteristics, and not permissible at a later stage where there are many more of these characteristics.

These decisions about selective termination of pregnancy in the presence of congenital disease are taken not just in the knowledge of their ethical permissibility, but also within the law of the relevant country. In the UK, termination of pregnancy is lawful if there is serious handicap at any stage of pregnancy. Abortion became legal under statute in 1967, and was modified slightly in 1990 by the Human Fertilisation and Embryology Act to the situation as described above.[29]

In some jurisdictions, abortion continues to be unlawful even in the presence of congenital disease, and in others, there are more restrictions than in the UK.

Summary

This chapter has reviewed the various conditions that the primary care practitioner might encounter in the area of genetic and congenital disease, as well as the screening programmes that are being developed and implemented. With the implementation of national screening programmes, it is clear that the primary health care professional will be faced with patients who are concerned about their screening result and the implications of their newborn for themselves. Clearly there is a need to increase genetic awareness through education and guideline development. Similarly, with the advent of IVF technology, there are bound to be ethical debates about reproductive decisions that will be challenging for practitioner and patient alike.

References

1. Newborn Screening Programme. *Polices and Standards for Newborn Blood Spot Screening.* London: Newborn Screening Programme; 2005.

2. Rosenstein BJ, Cutting GR. The diagnosis of cystic fibrosis: a consensus statement. *J Pediatr.* 1998; **132:** 589–95.

3. Rosentein BJ, Cutting GR. The diagnosis of cystic fibrosis: a consensus statement. *J Paediatr.* 1998; **132:** 589–95.

4. For further information, see www.newbornscreening-bloodspot.org.uk 18/05/07.

5. UK Collaborative Study of Newborn Screening (2004). Centre for Paediatric Epidemiology and Biostatistics. http://www.library.nhs.uk/SpecialistLibrarySearch/Download.aspx?resID=63577. (accessed 20th May 2007).

6. Davis A *et al.* A critical review of the role of neonatal hearing screening in the detection of congenital hearing impairment. *Health Technol Assess.* 1997; **1:** 1–176.

7. Deafness and hereditary hearing loss: overview. *GeneReviews*; www.genetests.org (accessed 21 February 2007).

8. Bitner-Glindzicz M. *Genetics and How it Relates to Newborn Hearing Screening.* London: Institute of Child Health and Great Ormond Street Hospital, Centre for Auditory Research; 2006.

9. Davies SC, Cronin E, Gill M *et al.* Screening for sickle-cell disease and thalassaemia: a systematic review with supplementary research. *Health Technol Assess.* 2000; **4:** 1–99.

10. Kai J, editor. *Antenatal and Newborn Screening Programmes: PEGASUS for front-line professionals. Education and training for genetic assessment manual. Version 1.5.2.* University of Nottingham; 2006.

11. See Chapter 8.

12. Weatherall D. Single gene disorders or complex traits: lessons from the thalassaemias and other monogenic disease. *BMJ.* 2000; **321:** 1117–20.

13. Committee of Enquiry into Human Fertilisation and Embryology; www.bopcris.ac.uk/bopall/ref21165.html 30.11.06.

14. Human Fertilisation and Embryology Authority Corporate Plan; www.hfea.gov.uk/cps/rde/xbcr/SID-3F57D79B-272CC6C7/hfea/The_HFEA_Corporate_plan_2004-2009.pdf (accessed 20 November 2006). This very readable document sets out plans for the next few years.

15. For a full account of its functions, which started in 1995, see www.ita.org.au (accessed 20 November 2006).

16. See www.agence-biomedecine.fr/fr/index.asp (with an English translation option) (accessed 20 November 2006). This body unifies all regulation for organ donation, reproduction, embryology and genetics – uniquely in Europe.

17. Chang WY, DeCherney AH. History of regulation of assisted reproduction technologies (ART) in the USA: a work in progress. *Hum Fertil.* 2003; **6:** 64–70. This article provides an overview of the American state of affairs.

18. Human Genetics Commission. *Making Babies: reproductive decisions and genetic technologies;* www.hgc.gov.uk/UploadDocs/DocPub/Document/Making%20Babies%20Report%20-%20final%20pdf.pdf 30.11.06.

19. Delhanty JDA. β-Thalassaemia: foetal HLA typing. *Lancet.* 2003; **363:** 6.

20. Sermon K, Steirteghem A, Liebaers I. Preimplanation genetic diagnosis. *Lancet.* 2004; **363:** 1633–40.

21. Genetics Commissioning Advisory Group, Department of Health. *Preimplantation Genetic Diagnosis (PGD): guiding principles for commissioners of NHS services.* London: Department of Health; 2002.

22. Magnus D, Caplan A. What is immoral about eugenics? *BMJ.* 1999; **319:** 1284–5.

23. Duncan RE, Foddy B, Delatycki M. Refusing to provide a genetic test: can it ever be ethical? *BMJ.* 2006; **333:** 1066–8.

24. Shakespeare T. Rights of future children. *BMJ.* 2006; **333:** 1173–4. Responses to Duncan *et al.* are included in the same volume, which also includes other useful commentary.

25. For a full explanation of this term, and an even more detailed explanation of this area, see Heyd D. Wrongful life: a pure genesis problem. In: *Genethics: moral issues in the creation of people.* Berkeley, CA: University of California Press; 1992.

26. Beauchamp T, Childress J. *Principles of Biomedical Ethics.* 3rd ed. Oxford: Oxford University Press; 1989. Beneficence as a moral principle in health care was first clearly described by Beauchamp and Childress in this book.

27. See two fine articles from the *Journal of Medical Ethics* for more detail: Herissone-Kelly P. Procreative beneficence and the prospective parent. *J Med Ethics.* 2006; **32:** 166–9 and Savulescu J. Procreative beneficence: why we should select the best children. *J Med Ethics.* 2001; **15:** 413–26.

28. See www.bcodp.org.uk/about/genetics.shtml for a full statement of this point.

29. The Abortion Act 1967 clarified the grounds for lawful termination of pregnancy in the UK. The Human Fertilisation and Embryology Act 1990 brought in some restrictions, but maintained the lawful basis of termination throughout pregnancy in the case of serious physical or mental handicap.

4

Exemplar genetic disorders

Introduction

Chapter 1 introduced the basic concept of inheritance and the possible modes of transmission of genetic disorders. The discussion in Chapter 3 focused on examples of screening genetic conditions which occur early on in life. This chapter will consider exemplar genetic conditions that may be managed in primary care, and in particular examples of late-onset genetic conditions which may illustrate the concept of a *monogenic* disorder.

The disorders that have been chosen will give an outline of some of the problems that are encountered when dealing with late-onset disorders, where although the genotype may be determined, there may be difficulties in determining when, if ever, there will be phenotypic expression – as in the case of haemochromatosis.

A good example of a late-onset disorder with the possibility of pre-symptomatic genetic testing is the case of Huntington's disease. Once an individual is diagnosed, there may well be implications for the rest of the family, and the principles of *cascade testing* of relatives are used. These principles will be discussed using myotonic dystrophy and familial hypercholesterolaemia as examples, whereby first-degree relatives of the affected individual may be tested.

Multifactorial conditions, where the interplay between environment and genetics plays a major role, are conditions encountered by primary care on a day-to-day basis, and examples of chronic common conditions, such as diabetes, heart disease and allergy, will be described later.

Autosomal dominant conditions

Box 4.1 Autosomal dominant conditions: examples

Adult polycystic renal disease
Familial hypercholesterolaemia
Huntington's disease
Neurofibromatosis type 1
Myotonic muscular dystrophy

Box 4.2 Autosomal dominant conditions: key points

Both males and females are affected.
The condition is manifested down through the generations.
There may be male-to-male transmission.
Homozygotes may be more severely affected than heterozygotes.
Presentation may occur as a late-onset disease.
Penetrance may vary in different individuals.

Adult polycystic renal disease[1]

Autosomal dominant polycystic kidney disease (ADPKD) is a disorder which has an onset in later life, with a 50% risk to the offspring of an affected parent. *De-novo* mutations may occur. It is characterised by renal cysts. Patients may present with recurrent urinary tract infections, haematuria and loin pain. The progressive renal damage can lead to hypertension. Cysts are found in other organs, including the pancreas and liver. The disorder is associated with vascular abnormalities, including intracranial aneurysms in 10% of affected individuals (a family history of subarachnoid haemorrhage may be present), mitral valve prolapse, aortic root dilatation and thoracic aortic dissections. By the age of 60 years, more than half of affected individuals may have end-stage renal disease (ESRD). Autosomal recessive polycystic kidney disease causes severe disease in infancy and early childhood, with affected individuals having enlarged kidneys and liver fibrosis. It may be detected by the antenatal ultrasound scan.

Alterations in the *PKD1* gene account for 85% of affected cases, whereas alterations in *PKD2* account for 15% of cases. *De-novo* mutations may occur in 10% of affected individuals. Patients with altered *PKD2* genes generally have less serious complications and a longer survival rate. Renal ultrasound is the main form of predictive testing, but genetic analysis of the PKD gene is possible in pre-symptomatic individuals. Prenatal testing is possible by chorionic villus sampling. However, it is rarely done because this is a late-onset genetic disorder.

Renal ultrasound scan in the third decade can be diagnostic, and the criteria for diagnosis are dependent on age. Thus under the age of 30 years there should be at least two unilateral or bilateral cysts, between 30 and 59 years there should be at least two cysts in each kidney, and after the age of 60 years there should be at least four cysts in each kidney.

The mainstay of management in primary care (with the involvement of the renal clinic) is the control of hypertension and renal failure and the prevention of extra-renal complications. Other cardiovascular factors need to be controlled in order to prevent renal failure, including the management of hyperlipidaemia. Cyst pain and haematuria are common, and analgesia is important. In pregnant women with ADPKD, the prevention of maternal and fetal complications is paramount through good blood pressure control.

For individuals who are concerned about their family history, the principles of diagnosis include assessing the kidneys for the presence of cysts using abdominal ultrasound, computed tomography (CT) or magnetic resonance imaging (MRI) scanning. If the diagnosis is unclear but the index of suspicion is high enough, genetic testing through a genetics centre would be the next step. If there is an affected parent, the risk to siblings of the index case is 50%. If the parents are unaffected, it is likely to be a *de-novo* mutation, and the risk to siblings is then much lower. Clearly patient education will be important, and the role of primary care is to ensure that patients are aware of the need for follow-up.

Familial hypercholesterolaemia

A question commonly asked by primary care clinicians is whether there is a family history of heart disease. A frequent biochemical test that is subsequently ordered, particularly if there is a positive response, is assessment of serum cholesterol and lipids. Patients have increasingly been proactive in requesting this, particularly if a family member has made it known that their cholesterol level is raised. Another factor in the UK that has made lipid measurements increasingly relevant is the Quality and Outcomes Framework (QOF). In general practice, registers have been set up to aid the assessment and management of patients with known coronary heart disease or diabetes.

There are some genetic disorders which can lead to abnormal lipid profiles, and perhaps the best known in general practice is familial hypercholesterolaemia. This is an autosomal dominant condition which is caused by mutations in the low-density-lipoprotein receptor (LDLR). In Europe, 1 in 500 of the population may be heterozygous for the LDLR mutation, which is the commoner form of familial hypercholesterolaemia found in general practice.

During the clinical assessment of such patients, it is important to enquire about early history of ischaemic heart disease (i.e. under 50 years in males and under 60 years in females). Clinical examination may reveal tendon xanthomata, which are firm swellings over tendons such as the Achilles tendon or tendons over knuckles, and arcus senilis.

In heterozygotes, cholesterol levels may be elevated from an early age, and by adulthood they may be in the range 9.0–14.0 mmol/l. These people are clearly at high risk of developing heart disease.

The Simon Broome Register Group[2] defines familial hypercholesterolaemia as a cholesterol level of >6.7 mmol/l in children under 16 years or >7.7 mmol/l in adults, plus tendon xanthomata in the patient (or a first- or second-degree relative of the patient).

The usual scenario faced by the GP is whether a patient with a high cholesterol level who does not fulfil the criteria is a possible case of familial hypercholesterolaemia. Obviously it is important to give lifestyle advice to patients, but statins are the mainstay of treatment. These are given from the late teens for men, and after completion of childbearing in women. Genetic mutations are identified by molecular genetic testing.

Cascade screening projects looking at how to identify family members through affected relatives have been initiated in the UK and particularly in the Netherlands.[3]

Huntington's disease

Huntington's disease has a prevalence of 7 in 100,000 in western European populations, although in certain subpopulations the prevalence has been found to be as high as 15 per 100,000. The disease is characterised by a progressive neurological condition that leads to a chorea movement disorder with intellectual impairment, psychiatric manifestations and dementia. It is predominantly an adult-onset disease, with an average age of diagnosis in the fifth decade. There is no treatment for this disease, and the median survival time is around 15 years. There is a rarer juvenile form which presents under the age of 20 years. Other differential diseases to consider include Parkinson's disease and Wilson's disease.

Huntington's disease is inherited in an autosomal dominant manner, and penetrance is almost 100%. The Huntington gene has been localised to the short arm of chromosome 4, and has been shown to be caused by an expansion of triplet CAG polyglutamine repeat sequences. Anticipation, whereby the onset of the disease occurs at an earlier age in succeeding generations, occurs where there is an increased number of repeat sequences and accounts for the juvenile form, which is characterised by more than 60 repeat sequences. Family members with an affected first-degree relative can receive predictive counselling, which requires expert genetic counselling both before and after testing. Genetic testing of asymptomatic children at risk is rarely undertaken. Similarly, although prenatal testing is possible, this is rarely done. Carriers of this altered gene require emotional and psychological support, which can be provided both by the genetic counsellors and by primary care physicians.

Neurofibromatosis

This is an autosomal dominant condition with a high *de-novo* mutation rate (i.e. the rate of development of a new mutation can be as high as 50%). The NF1 gene is important in cell growth and acts as a tumour suppressor. It is a condition that is characterised by variable expressivity of the disease that may be age dependent. This means that affected family members may express varying disease severity. In particular, there may be affected individuals who manifest very sporadic features with subtle disease. The birth incidence is around 1 in 3,000.

Clinical features include the presence of café au lait spots, which are brown macules found on the skin. These develop from infancy through childhood, and at least six café au lait spots of diameter 5 mm or more are necessary to support the diagnosis. Neurofibromata, which are tumours of neuro-fibrous tissue, may be found either in the superficial layers of the skin or in the more diffuse, deeper layers, as in plexiform neurofibromata. The latter may be found in early childhood, whereas the cutaneous forms usually develop through puberty. Other features include freckling in the axilla, optic gliomata, naevi in the iris known as Lisch nodules, and bony lesions including sphenoidal bone dysplasia. The diagnosis of NF1 requires the presence of at least two of the criteria listed in Box 4.3.[4]

Box 4.3 Clinical criteria for diagnosis of NF1

The diagnosis is clinically based on the presence of at least two of the following:

- six or more café au lait spots of diameter 5 mm or more in children and 15 mm or more in adults
- one or more plexiform neurofibromata, or two or more neurofibromata, including the cutaneous neurofibromata
- freckles on the axillae; other areas include the neck and the inguinal area
- two or more Lisch nodules
- thinning of the long bones or dysplasia of the sphenoid
- a sister, brother, child or parent with NF1.

Complications include developmental delay, particularly with difficulty in visuospatial awareness, spinal scoliosis, and the possibility of malignancy in the optic nerve, spine or soft tissues, renal artery stenosis and phaeochromocytoma.

In uncomplicated cases, annual follow-up may be undertaken by a paediatrician in childhood, and within primary care in adulthood, checking for complications, monitoring blood pressure and ensuring ophthalmology review. The involvement of the geneticist is important when reproductive advice is sought, or if there are features causing concern where multidisciplinary team involvement is necessary.

Myotonic dystrophy (MD)

The incidence of MD is around 1 in 8,000. Adults may present with weakness of the limbs, which may slowly progress with the presence of myotonia. It is an autosomal dominant condition which demonstrates anticipation. The alteration in the myotonica protein kinase gene is a repeating triplet sequence, and the number of repeats correlates with disease severity. Cascade family screening is an appropriate method of follow-up. This method relies on testing the index case and then following up relatives of the index case, usually starting with first-degree relatives.

The disease varies in its severity, and there is a congenital, more severe form, with babies presenting with hypotonia and respiratory distress. Typical clinical features in adults include daytime somnolence and fatigue, cardiac conduction defects, frontal balding, an increased risk of diabetes and cataracts. The myotonia may present with the patient's hand release being delayed (e.g. after hand shaking). There is an increased sensitivity to anaesthetics, sedatives and opiates. Adults may present between 20 and 30 years of age. In couples who are considering conception, pre-implanation diagnosis is available using DNA testing for the altered gene. Prenatal diagnosis is also available.

In females affected with myotonic dystrophy there are many potential obstetric complications, including prematurity.

MD is a disorder that could well be followed up in primary care. Patients need an annual ECG to exclude cardiac conduction defects, including a prolonged PR interval, as well as annual blood glucose tests to exclude diabetes.

Autosomal recessive conditions

Box 4.4 Autosomal recessive conditions: examples

Alpha-1-antitrypsin deficiency
Gilbert's syndrome
Haemochromatosis
Phenylketonuria
(For cystic fibrosis, sickle-cell disease and thalassaemia, *see* Chapter 3)

Box 4.5 Autosomal recessive conditions: key points

Both males and females are affected.
The disease is expressed in homozygotes only.
There is a 25% chance that a child will be affected if both parents are carriers.
These conditions are more common in consanguineous and ethnic groups.
There is seldom a positive family history except in consanguineous populations.

Alpha-1-antitrypsin deficiency

Lung connective tissue can be damaged by elastase, which is released by leucocytes. Alpha-1-antitrypsin is a protein that protects connective tissue from the harmful effects of elastase. Deficiency of this protein is an autosomal recessive condition with the gene encoding α-1-antitrypsin on chromosome 14. Deficiency leads to emphysema and liver disease, including cirrhosis. Gene mutations lead to impaired intracellular processing. Diagnosis of α-1-antitrypsin deficiency occurs by demonstrating low plasma concentrations of α-1-antitrypsin. Protease inhibitor (PI) typing or demonstrating mutations in the *SERPINA1* gene which codes for α-1-antitrypsin confirms the diagnosis.

As it is an autosomal recessive disorder, if both parents carry an altered gene, each sibling has a 25% chance of being affected, a 25% chance of being unaffected and a 50% chance of being a carrier. Testing for carrier status can be done by PI typing or mutation analysis for siblings and offspring of affected individuals.

The wild-type variant is known as M, the S variant is associated with a 40% reduction in plasma α-1-antitrypsin levels in homozygotes, and the Z variant is associated with an 85% reduction in plasma α-1-antitrypsin levels in homozygotes. PiM is the normal pattern, with 10% of European people being carriers for the S or Z variant.

Childhood-onset liver disease in individuals with PI ZZ may occur in a small number of affected individuals. Prenatal diagnosis is possible by genotyping parents' DNA from chorionic villus sampling.

It is important to advise individuals who are affected not to smoke, and to avoid occupations that involve exposure to environmental toxins.

In ZZ smokers there is double the loss of FEV1 (FEV1 is the volume of air exhaled during the first second of a forced exhalation) each year compared with unaffected non-smokers.

Surveillance is key to detecting deteriorating liver function, and monitoring of bilirubin, liver enzymes and clotting is important. Lung function tests, including spirometry, are recommended and can be performed in primary care if facilities are available.[5]

Gilbert's syndrome

Gilbert's syndrome is a common genetic disorder caused by a deficiency of the enzyme UDP-glucuronyl transferase, which leads to an increase in the levels of unconjugated bilirubin. Inheritance tends to follow an autosomal recessive pattern. Patients may present with mild jaundice, particularly at times of inter-current illness. Liver tests are otherwise normal. As much as 5% of the population may be affected, and the disorder is more common in males. It is a harmless benign condition.

Haemochromatosis

Haemochromatosis is an inherited autosomal recessive disorder that leads to organ damage due to excessive absorption of gastrointestinal iron. It may present with lethargy, painful joints and abdominal pain. The classic grey skin pigmentation indicates iron deposition in the skin, and other physical manifestations include hepatomegaly, testicular atrophy and swollen joints. The underlying condition arises because of iron depositions in major organs such as the liver, heart, pancreas, skin and other organs. The disease may be suspected if a middle-aged man presents with the rather vague symptoms described above. It may be confused with alcoholic cirrhosis. Untreated iron overload in the liver leads to cirrhosis and ultimately liver failure, together with hepatocellular cancer. Other complications include new-onset secondary diabetes mellitus, cardiac failure and arthritis. The onset of the disease typically occurs between the ages of 30 and 60 years. People who have demonstrable iron overload may require weekly venesection.

The HFE gene is found on 6p21. The two commonest alterations in the gene are C282Y and H63D caused by amino acid substitutions. Individuals may be homozygous or heterozygous for either, or they may be compound heterozygous, where there are different altered genes on each chromosome. There is ethnic variation, with alterations in the C282Y gene predominating in Celts but not usually in Asians. The factor that determines whether there are clinical symptoms associated with the alterations in the genes is the penetrance, and often it is incomplete, which means that although individuals may be carriers for the disease, they may never develop clinically significant disease. For example, in individuals who are homozygous for C282Y, penetrance may be as low as 1–5% in the general population, and higher in family members who may be at risk through an affected relative.

Investigations include liver function tests, and measurement of serum iron, ferritin and transferrin saturation. DNA tests include genotyping for C282Y and H63D. Further clinical investigations (e.g. hormone profiles) are indicated if clinical features are present. Liver biopsy may be indicated if there is a high ferritin level (e.g. >1,000 µg/l) or if liver function tests are abnormal.

Predictive testing is available. If there is an affected relative, first-degree relatives would be offered testing. If an individual is a carrier, their partner would be tested. Testing would be by genotyping and measurement of ferritin and transferrin levels. In the general population there is a 1 in 10 carrier risk. If the partner is not a carrier, the offspring are unlikely to develop disease. Monitoring of iron studies need to be measured annually in homozygotes, and this should be done annually.

Phenylketonuria

This condition is an example of an autosomal recessive condition that causes a biochemical disorder of amino acid metabolism (i.e. an inborn error of metabolism). The underlying problem is a deficiency of phenylalanine hydroxylase, an enzyme that plays an important part in the conversion of phenylalanine to tyrosine. The two effects are a build-up of phenylalanine, which if left untreated in children can lead to severe mental retardation, and epilepsy. Phenylalanine is converted to metabolites such as phenylpyruvic acid, which are toxic and are excreted in the urine. Blocking of the production of tyrosine, which is important for melanin production, can lead to affected children presenting with an albinoid-type syndrome.

The Guthrie heel prick test, which is performed on day 6 of life in neonates, is used to screen for phenlyketonuria. This condition is treated by restricting the dietary intake of phenylalanine, which has been shown to reduce the risk of mental retardation. The current recommendation is that the special diet should be continued indefinitely, partly because of the risk to the children of affected mothers.

X-linked conditions

Box 4.6 X-linked conditions: examples

Duchenne muscular dystrophy
Fragile X syndrome
Haemophilia A and B

Box 4.7 X-linked conditions: key points

X-linked dominant
Females usually express disease.
Lethal in males.
Multiple miscarriages.
There is no male-to-male transmission.
X-linked recessive
Males are affected.
Females are usually affected less severely.
There is no male-to-male transmission.

Duchenne muscular dystrophy

This hereditary muscular dystrophy is an X-linked recessive condition that affects males. It has an incidence of 1 in 3,500 males, with 1 in 2,500 females being carriers. It is characterised by a progressive muscle weakness that affects boys from the age of 3 to 5 years in 90% of cases. There is characteristic proximal muscle wasting and calf swelling, due to loss of muscle and its replacement by fat and connective tissue, resulting in affected boys being wheelchair bound by their early teens. The diagnosis should be considered in young boys when there is a developmental delay in speech or walking, with delays in motor milestones. Death commonly occurs before the second decade, due to cardiorespiratory failure.

The dystrophin gene that is found on the X chromosome is also transcribed in brain tissue, which accounts for learning difficulties in boys when there is alteration due to deletion of part of the gene. The protein produced by the gene is called dystrophin, and its absence leads to muscle cell degeneration.

Carriers of the altered gene can be biochemically tested by measuring creatinine kinase levels, which can be excessively high. Muscle biopsy can be diagnostic if DNA studies do not find an altered gene. However, DNA analysis together with creatinine kinase measurement will detect the majority of female carriers, and prenatal testing is available.

Fragile X syndrome

The main feature associated with fragile X syndrome is learning disability, including IQs as low as 40, associated with behavioural problems and/or autism. Clinical features include a long face, protruding ears, hypermobile joints, large testes and mitral valve prolapse. Males are commonly known to be affected, but females can be affected, too, although usually to a lesser degree. The genetic abnormality associated with this condition resides at a fragile area at the distal end of the X chromosome, where a dynamic triplet repeat mutation (CGG) has been found. In the UK, approximately 1 in 5,000 males carry the full mutation on the *FMR1* gene. In normal individuals, one would expect fewer than 45 repeats. In the pre-mutation carrier state, particularly in females, there are likely to be 55–200 repeats, whereas in affected individuals there are likely to be more than 200 repeats.

A DNA blood test is available which detects the altered gene, and various methods have been used to try to screen for fragile X syndrome, including cascade testing of relatives who might be at risk, and antenatal screening.[7] The risk is that the pre-mutation female carrier may pass on a full mutation to either a male or female offspring. This is dependent to some extent on the number of triplet repeats that the female carrier may have initially. A higher pre-mutation number of repeats has a greater chance of developing into the full mutation. Males with the pre-mutation will pass this on to all of their daughters and none of their sons. A quarter of all females who are pre-mutation carriers may develop premature menopause before the age of 40 years.

Affected individuals and their families may well need community paediatric support and special needs schooling. Complications include the development of cerebellar ataxia.

Haemophilia A and B

Haemophilia A is caused by a deficiency of factor VIII, which plays an important part in the intrinsic clotting pathway, whereby there is activation of prothrombin to thrombin, which converts fibrinogen to fibrin. The disease has an incidence of 1 in 5,000 males. Haemophilia B is caused by a deficiency of factor IX, and has an incidence of around 1 in 30,000. The severity of both conditions depends on the level of activity of factor VIII or IX, respectively. Haemophilia is a possible diagnosis if a male baby presents with multiple unexplained bruises, especially if there is a positive family history. The symptoms can range from relatively mild bleeding after dental treatment to spontaneous haemarthrosis. Both diseases are fully penetrant. Affected individuals are usually under the care of haematologists. They require follow-up to prevent complications, and advice on preparation for surgery and labour, and dealing with transfusion-related problems, including infection.

Chromosomal conditions

Down's syndrome

In trisomy 21 there are three copies of chromosome 21 per cell. The incidence of Down's syndrome is dependent on maternal age at delivery. For example, at the age of 30 years the incidence is 1 in 900, and this rises to 1 in 30 by the age of 45 years. The majority of cases occur because of *non-disjunction*. This is the process whereby failure of separation of homologous chromosomes at meiosis gives rise to daughter cells which may have one more or one less chromosome than normal.

The clinical characteristics include up-sloping palpebral fissures, small ears, tongue protrusion, single palmar creases, hypotonia and congenital cardiac malformations. Children usually have developmental delay, and in later life affected individuals may develop leukaemia or dementia.

In the UK, prenatal screening is used to look for a Down's affected fetus, which can include excess nuchal skin measured by ultrasound at 10–13 weeks' gestation. Increased fetal nuchal translucency is also detected in the presence of trisomy 13 (Patau's syndrome) and trisomy 18 (Edwards' syndrome), which are rare conditions, with most affected infants dying early. Other conditions, such as Turner's syndrome (see below), may also present with excess nuchal tissue.

The use of the triple test as a risk assessment at 14–16 weeks' gestation involves measurement of β-fetoprotein, β-human chorionic gonadotrophin and unconjugated oestriol. The quadruple test also includes inhibin A measurement. If the risk of a Down's baby is higher than 1 in 250, further testing by amniocentesis is necessary. Prenatal diagnosis is possible by chorionic villus sampling or amniocentesis, and the use of fluorescence *in situ* hybridisation (FISH) together with karyotyping has been the conventional investigation of choice. Aneuploidy exclusion using the quantitative fluorescent polymerase chain reaction (QF-PCR) alone for women found to be at increased risk of Down's syndrome is a rapid molecular test that is being introduced for women who have had a nationally approved Down syndrome screening test. The National Screening Committee policy position in July 2006 was that screening should be offered to all pregnant women, with the programme's national standards being as follows:

- a detection rate of at least 60% with a false-positive rate of 5% or less by 2004–5

- a detection rate of at least 75% with a false-positive rate of 3% or less by April 2007.

Recurrence rates tend to be low except in rare circumstances of chromosomal abnormalities.

Turner's syndrome

This syndrome is characterised by the karyotype 45X, where an absent X chromosome may be found in over 1 in 2,000 live female births. The clinical features associated with this condition include oedema of the hands or feet, short stature, a broad webbed neck, low hairline and ptosis. In as many as 50% of affected girls there may be abnormalities of the cardiovascular system, with aortic coarctation and ventricular septal defects. Abnormalities of the renal tracts also exist.

There may be delays in development, with delayed milestones and problems with social integration. Most women with Turner's syndrome are infertile. Girls with Turner's syndrome should be under the care of a specialist paediatrician during childhood, and a multidisciplinary team during adulthood. Development, particularly with regard to height, needs to be monitored, and appropriate treatment (e.g. growth hormone) initiated if indicated. Complications of Turner's syndrome include obesity, ovarian failure and deafness.

Cleft lip and palate

Cleft lip occurs due to failure of fusion of the primary palate, whereas cleft palate is due to failure of fusion of the secondary palate, during embryological development. The incidence of cleft lip, with or without cleft palate, in the general population is of the order of 1 in 1,000 births. Isolated cleft palate has an incidence of 4 in 10,000 births. It is important to exclude syndromic conditions that may have a cleft as a clinical finding. These include Van der Woude syndrome, which is an autosomal dominant condition, Pierre Robin sequence and associated trisomy 13 and 18. Anticonvulsant medication taken during pregnancy has also been implicated.

Isolated clefts are usually due to interplay between genetics and environment, and once syndromes and families with a clear inherited pattern have been excluded, it is possible to give recurrence risks to families who are concerned when a family member has been affected. The recurrence risk for a sibling affected with unilateral cleft lip and palate is 4%, compared with 2% for a sibling with isolated cleft lip. In isolated cleft palate, the recurrence risk is of the order of 2% with two affected siblings. Having an affected parent gives a recurrence risk of 4% for isolated cleft lip or palate.

It is possible to detect cleft lip at the 20-week gestation scan. However, small clefts may be missed, and cleft palate is difficult to detect at this stage. It is important that an expert multidisciplinary approach to the management of these affected families is adopted. In the UK, the Clinical Standards Advisory Group (CSAG) in its report on cleft lip and/or palate has stated that 'the experts for cleft lip and palate services should be concentrated within a small number of designated centres throughout the UK', and services have been organised in this way.

Conditions that have many causes

It is also the responsibility of the primary care team to care for patients whose illnesses are caused by a number of different mechanisms operating together. Much chronic disease occurs in this way.

It could be said that the aetiology of this kind of chronic disease is of little interest to the primary care practitioner, whose main concern is to minimise its effects, but that would be to belittle the larger picture within which patients consider their own illnesses. Diseases with many causes, otherwise known as multifactorial diseases, come in many different types, and a selection will now be considered.

Diabetes

Case study

C is a 48-year-old actuary. He attended a health screening appointment arranged through his employer, at which a large number of biochemical tests were performed. He was quite impressed with all this at the time, especially as it followed an exhaustive physical examination and history taking by the screening doctor. The only facts of any importance to emerge from all of this were his family history of type 2 diabetes (in his father and his paternal uncle), a high body mass index (BMI) and a fasting blood sugar level of 7.2 mmol/l.

C went to discuss this situation with his GP, handing over to her a 20-page printout of otherwise normal findings.

He was curious to know why he had these laboratory results.

Diabetes is a condition that is defined in biochemical terms as a fasting blood sugar level that is found to be over 7 mmol/l on several occasions. The potential adverse effects on long-term health do not need to be stated here.

Of the two types of diabetes mellitus, more than 75% of patients have type 2, or what used to be termed non-insulin-dependent diabetes. Box 4.8 summarises the factors known to be associated with the causation of type 2 diabetes.

Box 4.8 Causes of type 2 diabetes

• Increased sugar production in the liver
• Genetic factors
• Environmental factors
• Increased fat breakdown
• Abnormalities of insulin
• Altered gut hormones

Disentangling these causes is complicated in individual patients – and even more so when factors relating to genes and environment are involved. It is known that about 30% of patients with type 2 diabetes have a family member similarly affected, and this figure rises to 40% in the case of a first-degree relative. However, families often share the same patterns of diet and exercise, so identifying the exact cause is not easy.

The LpL gene has been associated with diabetes, and a genetic pattern for maturity-onset diabetes of youth (MODY) has been identified. In fact the latter is a rare example of a single-gene illness, in contrast to the more common varieties of type 2 diabetes, which are polygenic.

One of these variants has shown different responses to treatment. Those patients with the HNF-1β gene respond markedly better to sulphonylurea anti-diabetic drugs than do other type 2 patients.

In the case of type 1 diabetes, which accounts for slightly less than a quarter of cases, similar overlaps of environmental and hereditary factors are involved. The genetic abnormalities arise in various sites in the genome. The human lymphocyte antigen is an immune protein associated with damage to the β-pancreatic cells that produce insulin. The vast majority of Caucasian type 1 patients have either the HLA-DR3 or HLA-DR4 alleles.

Chromosome 11 contains the genes that code for insulin itself, and has also been implicated in the disease. In total, 18 regions of the genome have been studied in relation to type 1 diabetes.[10]

Arguably, what is of most interest to primary care is the interaction between genetic predisposition and environmental influence. Patients can change neither their families nor their genes, but they can change their behaviour in ways that can alter the progress or even the genesis of diabetes. This raises an intriguing dilemma for both clinician and patient: could it be said that a person at increased genetic risk of diabetes is under more of a responsibility to alter their behaviour in order to reduce their overall risk? The most important environmental risk factors in type 2 diabetes are obesity and physical inactivity. Overcoming these risks would lead to markedly less illness.

However, it is a large step to accord individuals responsibility for their illnesses because of their behaviour, and an even larger one to accord them increased responsibility if they are genetically more vulnerable.

As a new patient with (probable) type 2 diabetes, C will have many questions about his condition, and it is part of good primary care to offer explanation and education. C's professional occupation may lead him to a greater understanding of the risks of secondary complications of diabetes than is generally seen.

Ischaemic heart disease

Case study

D's wife attends her GP a few days after the sudden death of her husband, a 50-year-old plumber (a patient of the same GP). A post-mortem examination had revealed D's widespread coronary artery disease, of which he had little knowledge. The doctor took time to discuss D's wife's state of mind, and offered further help. Part of her grief centred on whether she might have prevented her husband's death.

Still the largest agent of early death in the western world, ischaemic heart disease (also known as IHD or coronary artery disease) is again an illness with many causes. As with diabetes, some of these factors can be modified by individual behaviour, and some cannot. The impact of the family history per se, although difficult to quantify, cannot be avoided.

Box 4.9 Causes of ischaemic heart disease

- Raised serum cholesterol level
- Smoking
- A family history of IHD
- Other pathology (e.g. diabetes)
- Excessive alcohol consumption

Family history must have a genetic basis, and in recent years the precise gene loci that engender a predisposition to IHD have been identified. For the most part these findings are still on a research footing and not generally available as screening or investigative tests.

In 1992, a group of Danish men with the Lewis blood group Le(a-b), expressed from chromosome 19, were found to have a higher risk of IHD.[11] Similar studies have found associations between early IHD and specific gene abnormalities, but this is still an emerging (and contested) field. For example, in 2003 an association was postulated between early IHD and the MEF2A gene. This 21-base-pair deletion (a mutation termed β7aa) had been found in a family in which every member had premature IHD. Later research on similar families in Japan and Ireland did not reproduce this finding, so the association between genetic and clinical factors remains unconfirmed.[12]

It remains important to consider the pathogenesis of IHD. The various risk factors listed above culminate in atherosclerosis of the coronary circulation, and a genetic influence can contribute at any stage of the process. Associations have been identified between the various lipoprotein lipase genotypes, higher serum lipid subfractions and IHD risk.[13]

Recently, one very interesting finding has drawn inferences about IHD in the general population from knowledge of the rare genetic disease homocystinuria. Patients with this disease have high homocysteine levels in the blood, and when prescribed the simple treatment of oral folic acid, their otherwise high rates of IHD are also reduced. It is postulated that the general population may benefit similarly, on epidemiological analysis.[14]

Research has also been done on the inflammatory processes now held to be of importance in the genesis of IHD, and each of these factors has increasing genetic relevance as research proceeds. However, the task for clinicians in primary care actually changes little, for the moment, from care of the individual patient who is subject to all of these influences.

Allergic disease

Case study

F is a 1-year-old child who has always suffered from infantile eczema. His parents regularly consult their NHS practice, as F needs continuous treatment with emollients, topical steroids and other interventions. Occasionally F's skin develops secondary infections, exacerbating the usual itching and inflammation of the skin. Recently, he has begun to have attacks of wheezing as well. F's father suffered similar but less intense symptoms in his own childhood.

Readers will be familiar with the spectrum of atopic disorders, including asthma, eczema and allergic rhinitis. The incidence of atopy, particularly in childhood, is surprisingly high, and prevalence rates of asthma are quoted as being around 10% in the UK. The prevalence in adults is around 5%, and this includes a proportion of non-atopic asthma.

Familial clustering of patients with atopic diseases occurs, but there is no single gene pattern or predictable inheritance pattern. Thus there is, as in the case of diabetes and IHD, a subtle interaction of environment and inheritance.

Recent research has begun to illuminate this interaction more fully.

First, the increasing prevalence of asthma suggests that changes in the environment may be interacting in a different way with genetic predispositions. For example, it has been suggested that our lessening contact with saprophytic organisms as a result of urbanisation somehow modulates immune responses such that greater allergy is a consequence.[15] Clearly, if this is true, it indicates a genetic 'preference' for more contact with the soil!

Secondly, the increasing prevalence of atopic disease does not seem to be a result of greater diagnostic awareness. In other words, health care professionals – and this may be of particular relevance to primary care – are not diagnosing these conditions more easily, or at a lower threshold. The prevalence change is real.[16]

Thirdly, the precise gene loci implicated in allergic disease are being identified, and it seems that some genes represent vulnerabilities and others represent protective qualities.

Box 4.10 Gene loci associated with allergic disease[17]

Chromosome 5: interleukins 3, 5, 9 and 13
Chromosome 11: β-chain of high-affinity IgE receptor
Chromosome 16: IL-4 receptor
Chromosome 12: stem-cell factor, interferon β, etc.

The future implications of this research are that groups at risk for allergy might potentially be identified in childhood, with the possibility of early intervention by way of treatment. In addition, in the long term there is the possibility of curative genetic therapy.

Familial clustering, and by implication genetic loading, is seen in drug hypersensitivity, too. Patients are often very aware of a family history of drug allergy, and keen to make their primary care teams similarly aware. This is an area fraught with clinical difficulty in view of the imprecision associated with the diagnosis of drug allergy or intolerance.[18] Specific gene loci have been identified in the HLA system. For example, HLA DR-3 is associated with hypersensitivity to gold, and there are other relationships. The mechanism at work here is a double-edged sword, as it hinges on a drug being recognised as foreign or antigenic. Ostensibly this is protective, but it actually leads to hypersensitivity manifestations.[19]

In the future, it may become possible to link individual hypersensitivity to particular parts of individual genomes, thereby predicting the clinical consequences.

Dementia

Alzheimer's disease is characterised by pathological amyloid deposits in neurofibrillary tangles and extracellular amyloid senile plaques. It is the commonest cause of both presenile (<60 years of age) and senile (>60 years) dementia. Clinically, with normal consciousness, there is a global, progressive and irreversible impairment of social skills, memory and intellectual capacity, together with emotional lability. In just under 50% of cases, apolipoprotein E is found in neuronal plaques, and it is considered to be a risk factor for the development of late-onset dementia, with genetic testing being of limited value.

Dementia is also associated with other genetic disorders, such as Huntington's disease. Autosomal dominant fronto-temporal dementia is associated with Parkinson's disease. Dementia caused by repeated strokes due to vascular disorders tends to be multifactorial in nature. Early-onset dementia does require assessment by a specialist physician.[1]

Risk assessment and consequences

The discussion of these various diseases thus far has rather inadequately considered the notion of risk itself.

In the above section, each of the factors determining disease outcome can be allocated a quantitative risk based on current knowledge. In the case of IHD, clinicians can refer to resources such as the New Zealand[20] or Framingham[21] tables – risk factors for individual patients can be taken together and an individualised risk calculated. It helps both clinician and patient to decide whether, for example, a statin could be useful, effective and relevant. In neither of these resources are family history and therefore genetic loading included in the calculation, but they may be involved in the discussion about the mathematical risk. To that extent, the additional risk posed by a family history is a matter of professional judgement for the clinician and of autonomous decision making for the patient.

The larger issue in any discussion of risk in general, or of genetic risk in particular, is the way in which this kind of information is handled, processed and understood by patients. Genetic counselling often includes a mathematical assessment of risk – communicated to a patient and their family – of a genetic 'event.' As such, it is similar to the kind of discussion that a clinician might have with a patient about cardiovascular risk.

However, there is evidence that patients can find numerical risk difficult to handle, process or understand, and that clinicians need to find creative ways of having this discussion. Several authors have argued that professionals need to

find ways of reinterpreting data with patients to make their level of understanding more complete, perhaps by using pictorial representations[22] or standar-
dising the language of risk. For example, perhaps 'high' should always mean a
risk of less than 1 in 100 and 'moderate' should always mean a risk of between
1 in 1,000 and 1 in 100.[23] If this were to happen (a somewhat unlikely prospect),
clinicians and patients might at least achieve a common language of risk.

In the case of much of the pathology that has been dealt with in this chapter,
there is an interaction between genetic risk and other factors (each with its own
risks). The necessary connection is the link between a patient understanding
these risks and their making behavioural changes as a result (e.g. refraining from
smoking or curtailing fatty food consumption). It is said that this connection
requires the strengthening of two beliefs or assumptions – first, that changing
behaviour can reduce the risk of serious consequences, and secondly, that there
is an ability to change behaviour.[24] Both of these beliefs can and should be
supported in primary care.

Summary

This chapter has illustrated numerous genetic conditions that may well be
encountered in primary care. These genetic conditions may range from
monogenic disorders with clear Mendelian inheritance patterns to multifactorial conditions that highlight the relationship and interplay between environment, lifestyle and genetics. The purpose of the chapter has been to introduce
some well-known genetic conditions and consider the management issues that
might be pertinent to primary care. Each genetic condition that a primary care
physician may encounter brings different challenges, which may include issues
relating to diagnosis, clinical management or genetic testing, and counselling
and the family, particularly in late-onset disorders.

References

1. Harris PC, Torres VE. Autosomal dominant polycystic kidney disease. *GeneReviews*;
   www.genetests.org (accessed 31 January 2007).

2. Steering Committee of the Simon Broome Register Group. Risk of fatal coronary
   heart disease in familial hypercholesterolaemia. *BMJ.* 1991; **303**: 893–6.

3. Austin MA *et al.* Familial hypercholesterolemia and coronary heart disease: a HuGE
   Association review. *Am J Epidemiol.* 2004; **160**: 421–9.

4. National Institutes of Health Consensus Development Conference.
   Neurofibromatosis. Conference statement. *Arch Neurol.* 1988; **45**: 575–8.

5. Schlade-Bartusiak K, Cox DW. Alpha-1-antitrypsin deficiency. *GeneReviews*;
   www.genetests.org (accessed 28 October 2006).

6. Barnicoat A. Screening for fragile X syndrome: a model for genetic disorders? *BMJ.*
   1997; **315**: 1174–5.

7. Public Health Genetics Unit. Fragile X syndrome; www://phgu.org.uk/pages/info/
   diseases/fragilex.htm (accessed 11 February 2007).

8. UK Clinical Standards Advisory Group; www.dh.gov.uk/PolicyAndGuidance/Health AndSocialCareTopics/SpecialisedServicesDefinition/SpecialisedServicesDefinitionArti cle/fs/en?CONTENT_ID=4001685&chk=jLwtjp (accessed 3 March 2007).

9. Pearson ER *et al.* Genetic cause of hyperglycaemia and response to treatment in diabetes. *Lancet.* 2003; **362:** 1275–81.

10. A full report from the World Health Organization can be found at www.who.int/genomics/about/Diabetis-fin.pdf 1.12.06.

11. Hein HO *et al.* The Lewis blood group: a new marker of genetic disease. *J Intern Med.* 1992; **6:** 481–7.

12. Horan PG, Allen AR *et al.* Lack of MEF2A β7aa mutation in Irish families with early-onset ischaemic heart disease: a family-based study. *BMC Med Genet.* 2006; **7:** 65.

13. Wittrup HH, Andersen RV *et al.* Combined analysis of six lipoprotein lipase genetic variants on triglycerides, high-density lipoprotein, and ischemic heart disease: cross-sectional, prospective, and case–control studies from the Copenhagen City Heart Study. *J Clin Endocrinol Metab.* 2006; **91:** 1438–45.

14. Wald DS, Morris JK *et al.* Folic acid, homocysteine and cardiovascular disease: judging causality in the face of inconclusive trial evidence. *BMJ.* 2006; **333:** 1114–7.

15. von Hertzen L, Haahtela T. Disconnection of man and the soil: a reason for the asthma and atopy epidemic. *J Allergy Clin Immunol.* 2006; **117:** 334–44.

16. Upton MN, McConnachie A *et al.* Intergenerational 20-year trends in the prevalence of asthma and hay fever in adults: the Midspan family study surveys of parents and offspring. *BMJ.* 2000; **328:** 88–92.

17. Borish L. Genetics of allergy and asthma. *Ann Allergy Asthma Immunol.* 1999; **82:** 413–26.

18. Pirmohamed M. Genetic factors in the predisposition to drug-induced hypersensitivity reactions. *AAPS Journal.* 2006; **8:** Article 3.

19. Ibid.

20. Oxford Evidence-Based Medicine Centre; www.cebm.net/prognosis.asp 1.12.06.

21. Framingham CHD calculator; www.patient.co.uk/showdoc/40000133 1.12.06.

22. Edwards A, Elwyn G, Mulley A. Explaining risks: turning numerical data into meaningful pictures. *BMJ.* 2002; **324:** 827–30.

23. Calman K, Royston G. Risk language and dialects. *BMJ.* 1997; **315:** 939–42.

24. Marteau TM, Lerman C. Genetic risk and behavioural change. *BMJ.* 2001; **322:** 1056–9.

5

Cancer genetics

Introduction

Perhaps the largest numbers of referrals that are received by a genetics department from primary care are those relating to cancer genetics. Patients who are concerned about their cancer risk based on their family history may be seeking genetic counselling, screening advice or consideration for genetic testing.

Ideally, the role of primary care should be to reassure the low-risk families while seeking advice from the regional genetic centre about high-risk groups. In the UK, there are service development pilots which are assessing the role of the genetics nurse counsellor in running clinics in the community for this purpose.[1] The Department of Health has also funded 10 GPs with a specialist interest in genetics. Most are promoting the concept of primary care genetics through education and, in one or two instances, through service development.

The commonest histories of people evaluated through cancer genetics clinics are those relating to bowel and breast cancer. Clinical screening and surveillance are important measures that need to be understood in order to allow an informed discussion on management options. This chapter will consider some of the commoner conditions encountered by both cancer geneticists and primary care physicians.

It is important to understand that most of the genes that increase susceptibility to cancer are inherited in an autosomal dominant manner (*see* Chapter 1). Thus in classic autosomal dominant inheritance patterns, altered cancer-causing genes may allow equal transmission by both sexes, there are no skipped generations, and each child has a 50% chance of inheriting the altered gene. However, factors that affect penetrance include the lifestyle–environment–genetic balance, and thus also influence the risk of developing cancer. Such factors include smoking and the influence of hormones.

Family history and the role of primary care

The essence of being able to give genetic advice or counselling is a detailed family history. It is important that all cancers affecting family members are noted, including the age of onset, the type of cancer, and the presence of unilateral or bilateral disease (as in the case of breast cancer) or multiple cancers in individuals. Extracolonic associations sometimes form syndromes in families affected by cancer. Clearly, taking a detailed family history is time consuming (*see* Box 5.1).

Verification of cancers by confirming the pathology details is important. Family members require counselling both about their own risk and also about the options available for surveillance and the relevance of genetic testing. This is particularly important in autosomal dominant cancer syndrome families.

Box 5.1 Taking the family history

It is useful to take a three-generation family history. In relation to breast cancer, it is important to ask about the ages at which relatives were diagnosed with breast and ovarian cancer, as well as the ages at which they died. Both female- and male-affected breast cancers should be recorded. It should also be documented whether there are cases where family members might have, or have had, bilateral breast cancers, ovarian cancers or other cancers (including uterine, colon and prostate cancer and melanoma).

Ethnic origin is relevant (e.g. recording whether there are family members of Jewish origin, particularly Ashkenazi Jews) (see later).

Information such as where the cancer was treated and what type of treatment was received will help to determine the reliability of the diagnosis. Verifying the family history confirms the patient's account, and the regional genetics unit frequently follows up on death certificates and pathology reports and seek further clarification from relatives before accepting that the family pedigree is correct.

Breast and ovarian cancer

Case 1

A 39-year-old woman attends her GP for a new patient registration. She mentions that her mother died of breast cancer at the age of 69 years, and asks if she is at increased risk of developing breast cancer herself.

Assuming that there is no other family cancer history, this woman should be reassured that her risk is close to the general population risk, and that her mother's cancer was probably sporadic. Breast cancer is common. In the UK, the lifetime risk of developing breast cancer is 1 in 9. Factors other than genetics that influence the risk of developing breast cancer include hormonal factors and environmental factors. Thus giving lifestyle advice such as encouraging the patient to take regular exercise, avoid obesity and drink alcohol only in moderation, and encouraging breastfeeding, is appropriate. Other factors that affect the breast cancer risk include the use of the oral contraceptive pill, hormone replacement therapy (HRT), early menarche or late menopause, having children late or not having children at all, and exposure to ionising radiation (e.g. women treated with mantle radiotherapy for lymphoma).[2]

The likelihood of carrying an altered dominant gene that predisposes to breast or ovarian cancer is increased if:

• the age of the affected family member is relatively young
• there are many affected family members
• within breast cancer families there are family members affected with ovarian cancer, especially if they are affected by both breast and ovarian cancer.

For example, if there is only one affected family member, the chances of finding an altered gene are remote, whereas if there are more than three affected family members with breast cancer on the same side of the family, the chances of finding an altered gene are high. The important point to note when making a risk assessment after taking a family history is to warn the consultand that their risk might change if other family members were to develop cancer. The presence of a male breast cancer is important because of its rarity, and increases the chance that it is genetic. Similarly, the presence of bilateral breast cancer in a close relative is significant, increasing the risk of an underlying genetic cause.

BRCA1 and BRCA2

Hereditary breast and ovarian cancer accounts for a small proportion (5–10%) of cases overall. The commonest breast cancer-causing genes are BRCA1 and BRCA2. Mutations or alterations in these genes are associated with a high risk of developing breast and ovarian cancer by an autosomal dominant mode of inheritance (*see* Box 5.2). Both BRCA1 and BRCA2 are large genes, and alterations in the coding sequence may be found throughout the gene. Both genes are important for normal DNA repair mechanisms. Mutations in the BRCA1 or BRCA2 genes account for more than 80% of autosomal dominant breast and ovarian cancer families. Alterations in the BRCA2 gene predispose men to breast cancer, with a 6% lifetime risk.

There are specific populations which have an increased risk of cancers, and these include the Ashkenazi Jewish population, particularly in Eastern Europe, who have an increased risk of developing BRCA1- and BRCA2-associated cancers.

Box 5.2 High-risk genes and associated cancers

	BRCA1	BRCA2
Lifetime risk:		
Breast cancer	60–90%	50–80%
Second primary breast cancer	60%	50%
Ovarian cancer	20–40%	20%

Patients with BRCA1 and BRCA2 mutations are at increased risk of developing other types of cancers. For example, carriers of a mutated BRCA2 gene have a relative risk of 4.65 (range 3.48–6.22) of developing prostate cancer.[3] However, screening programmes for these cancers have not been defined.

Li–Fraumeni syndrome

A further autosomal dominant condition that may predispose to cancers, including breast cancer, is the Li–Fraumeni syndrome. In affected family members there may be a range of tumour types at a young age, including breast cancer, sarcoma, brain tumours and adrenocortical cancers, and phyllodes (fibro-epithelial tumours). Other associated cancers include stomach and pancreatic cancers.

The syndrome is accounted for by an alteration in a tumour suppressor gene, TP53, which is important in cell cycle regulation. DNA analysis to detect alteration in the TP53 gene is available. The cancer risk is very high in carriers of an altered TP53 gene.

National Institute for Clinical Excellence (NICE) guidelines for familial breast cancer

Many guidelines, with regional variations, exist for the management of these patients – for example, the Cancer Research Campaign familial breast and ovarian cancer guidelines that were published in 2001 for primary care. However, the NICE guidelines for familial breast cancer are also relevant to primary care, and were updated in October 2006.[4]

These guidelines stipulate the need to give clear information to patients, to make a risk assessment and to be aware of local referral pathways. Table 5.1 indicates the level of thresholds, based on 10-year risk and lifetime risk status, in which women may fall into low-, moderate- or high-risk groups.

Table 5.1: Risk stratification for women aged 40–49 years

	10-year risk	Lifetime risk	Overall risk
Primary care	<3%	<17%	Low
Secondary care	3–8%	17–30%	Moderate
Tertiary care	>8%	>30%	High*

* Or >20% chance of an abnormal BRCA1, BRCA2 or TP53 gene.

We shall now consider a sequence of cancer genetics patient histories which refer to either moderate-risk or high-risk families. Referral criteria have been produced by NICE (see below). Referral could occur to secondary care breast clinics for breast screening, including the use of mammography, or to a tertiary regional genetics unit for consideration of genetic testing and genetic counselling.

Case 2

A 45-year-old woman is concerned about her family history. She has just found out that her sister has been diagnosed with breast cancer at the age of 53 years. Her mother had also been diagnosed with breast cancer, at the age of 59 years.

(In this case, there are two family members on the same side who have been diagnosed with breast cancer, with an average age of less than 60 years. Therefore the consultand is at moderate risk of developing breast cancer.)

Case 3

A 31-year-old woman has consulted her GP because she is aware that her sister has had breast cancer at the age of 39 years.

(In this case, a family member presents with breast cancer under the age of 40 years. Therefore the consultand is at moderate risk of developing breast cancer.)

Case 4

The sister of one of your patients wants to know her risk status after learning that her brother has been diagnosed with breast cancer at 59 years of age.

(In this case, there is significance attached to a male presenting with breast cancer. Breast cancer in males is rare, and accounts for less than 1% of all breast cancer cases, but it does confer a moderate risk for the consultand.)

Case 5

A 47-year-old woman is concerned about her family history. She is aware that her sister was diagnosed with breast cancer at the age of 53 years and with ovarian cancer at 57 years.

(The important facts in this case are the presence of two associated cancers. Breast cancer and ovarian cancers in the same family must raise awareness about the possibility that high-risk genes (e.g. BRCA 1) are present in the family. In the absence of any other family history this would fall in the moderate risk group for the consultand. However, if the sister presented with age at diagnosis of the first cancer under 50 years, this would be considered to be a high-risk family.)

Case 6

A 25-year-old woman seeks genetic counselling. Her sister had been diagnosed with breast cancer at the age of 29 years. Her mother had been diagnosed with ovarian cancer at 42 years of age, and a maternal aunt had been diagnosed with breast cancer at 37 years of age.

(In this case there is a chance of finding a family member who may carry an altered BRCA1 or BRCA2 gene. The main pointers are the fact that the affected family members are presenting at a young age, and the presence of both breast and ovarian cancer, with three family members affected. A referral to the local genetics clinic is needed.)

NICE referral criteria from primary to secondary care

The following referral criteria are based on NICE guidelines, and relate to individuals who may require more than reassurance, and need to be followed up in a breast clinic or family history clinic with relevant screening.

When taking a family history, it is important to note the following points.

- When guidance refers to relatives, these must be on the same side of the family and be blood relatives of the consultand and each other.
- Ethnicity is also an important factor to bear in mind, with Ashzenazi Jews being 5 to 10 times more likely to be carriers of the BRCA1 or BRCA2 gene mutations compared with the non-Jewish population.
- In women with bilateral breast cancer, each breast cancer has the same count as one relative.

Female breast cancers only

- One first-degree relative and one second-degree relative diagnosed before an average age of 50 years.
- Two first-degree relatives diagnosed before an average age of 50 years.
- Three or more first- or second-degree relatives diagnosed at any age.

Male breast cancer

One first-degree male relative diagnosed at any age.

Bilateral breast cancer

One first-degree relative where the first primary was diagnosed before the age of 50 years.

Breast and ovarian cancer

One first- or second-degree relative with ovarian cancer at any age and one first- or second-degree relative with breast cancer at any age (one should be a first-degree relative).

Referral from either primary or secondary care to tertiary (regional genetics unit)

The referral criteria below mainly relate to high-risk family members who may want to consider genetic testing or risk-reducing surgery.

Female breast cancers only

- Two first- or second-degree relatives diagnosed before an average age of 50 years, with at least one of them being a first-degree relative of the consultand.
- Three first- or second-degree relatives diagnosed before an average age of 60 years, with at least one of them being a first-degree relative of the consultand.
- Four relatives diagnosed at any age, with at least one of them being a first-degree relative of the consultand.

Ovarian cancer

- One relative diagnosed with ovarian cancer at any age and on the same side of the family.

- One first-degree relative (including a relative with ovarian cancer) or one second-degree relative diagnosed with breast cancer before the age of 50 years.
- One additional relative diagnosed with ovarian cancer at any age.
- Two first- or second-degree relatives diagnosed with breast cancer before an average age of 60 years.

Bilateral breast cancer

- One first-degree relative with cancer diagnosed in both breasts before the age of 50 years.
- One first- or second-degree relative diagnosed with bilateral breast cancer and one first- or second-degree relative diagnosed with breast cancer before an average age of 60 years.

Male breast cancer

- One male breast cancer diagnosed at any age and on the same side of the family.
- One first- or second-degree relative diagnosed with breast cancer before the age of 50 years.
- Two first- or second-degree relatives diagnosed with breast cancer before an average age of 60 years.

Screening and surveillance

In primary care, if a woman is deemed to be at low risk of developing breast or ovarian cancer based on her family history, some advice can be offered. It is important to warn the patient that if their family history changes, they will need to re-consult in order to re-evaluate their risk. They should be advised to be aware of any changes in their breast, including skin changes and nipple retraction or discharge. Lifestyle changes are relevant, with the need to avoid obesity and reduce alcohol intake, and breastfeeding should be encouraged. The relationship between breast cancer and duration of use of HRT and oral contraceptives should also be examined.

For women who are at increased risk of developing breast cancer, the same advice needs to be given, together with information about which appropriate screening options are available. An advantage of family history clinics for breast cancers is the multidisciplinary input into the care of such patients.

One decision that should be based on the family history is the type of surveillance necessary, and how often this would be required. In young women, breast tissue is dense, and this makes evaluation using standard mammography difficult. The exposure to radiation over many years that is necessary for long-term surveillance needs to be considered. There is a theoretical risk of inducing malignancy in women who are carrying an altered TP53 gene, if they are exposed to the radiation produced by mammography.

The NICE guidelines recommend annual MRI surveillance of the breasts in women aged 30–39 years who are at high risk and known to have a genetic mutation (i.e. BRCA1, BRCA2 or TP53). Similar surveillance is necessary for women aged 40–49 years who have a greater than 20% 10-year risk of developing breast cancer or a greater than 12% risk particularly if there is dense breast tissue on mammography. This has resource implications which regional genetics centres and radiology departments will need to consider, and around which they will need to plan MRI resource allocation.

Women for whom it has not been determined that they have a genetic mutation, but who on the basis of their family history have a greater than 30% risk of carrying the BRCA1 gene or an alteration in the TP53 gene, should be offered annual MRI surveillance from 30–49 years of age.

Women aged 40–49 years who have a moderately increased risk of developing breast cancer should have annual mammography, and then be included in the NHS breast-screening programme from the age of 50 years onwards. Family members may require more frequent screening after the age of 50 years, if they are deemed to be at high risk.

In disease surveillance for ovarian cancer, there are ongoing trials to assess the benefit of pelvic ultrasound and measurement of Cancer antigen 125 (CA125) blood levels. The UK Familial Ovarian Cancer Screening Study (UKFOCSS)[5] is currently assessing the value of annual pelvic ultrasound and CA125 blood levels in people with positive family histories.

Genetic counselling and gene testing in genetic units

In women who need predictive genetic testing, genetic counselling should be offered which covers the nature of hereditary breast and ovarian cancer, the purpose and interpretation of gene testing, and the implications. The protocol for testing involves testing an affected family member first.

When an alteration is identified in the relevant gene, this could then be used to offer testing for other family members. However, it has been shown that testing identifies an alteration in a gene in only 30% of families with affected family members where the risk is more than 20%. Female family members who are not found to be carrying an altered gene are deemed to have the general population level of risk of developing breast or ovarian cancer.

If an alteration in the breast-cancer-causing gene is not determined in affected individuals, then testing of other family members is not available and management should be according to family history.

Surgery: the role of prophylactic mastectomy and oophorectomy

Women who are considering risk-reducing surgery should be under the care of a specialist genetics centre. The options that are available to women who are at high risk of developing either breast cancer or ovarian cancer include bilateral mastectomy, and oophorectomy. A full risk assessment and verification of the family history is necessary. It is important that the counselling process is appropriate, and that a multidisciplinary team is involved in providing psychological support and assessment. Both types of surgery are offered to a small proportion of women at risk, carrying altered BRCA1, BRCA2 and TP53 genes.

Neither procedure completely eradicates the risk of disease. Prophylactic oophorectomy reduces the relative risk of breast cancer by up to 50% in families with known carriers of altered BRCA1 or BRCA2 genes, and reduces the risk of ovarian cancer by 95%. Bilateral mastectomy gives a relative risk reduction of 95% in the lifetime risk of developing breast cancer. Clearly, the potential complications of surgery and morbidity need to be taken into account, and women do need to be prepared psychologically prior to surgery.

Breast cancer risk factors in women with a positive family history

When advising women about HRT to counteract menopausal symptoms, they should be made aware that HRT use should be minimised because of the increase in breast cancer risk (particularly with more than 5 years' use of HRT). Similarly, although the oral contraceptive pill protects against ovarian cancer, there is an increase in breast cancer risk after the age of 35 years. General lifestyle advice includes weight reduction, avoidance of excessive alcohol intake, and attention to the benefits of exercise and breastfeeding.

Colorectal cancer

Introduction

There are approximately 30,000 cases per year and 15,000 deaths per year in the UK. This disease occurs more commonly in males than in females, with an age-standardised male:female ratio of 1.5:1. There is a transition from colonic mucosa tissue to adenoma (dysplastic or villous) formation and then to carcinoma, which involves a sequence of alterations in specific genes.[6]

The majority of bowel cancers are sporadic, caused by an interaction between lifestyle, environment and genetics. They commonly occur between 60 and 70 years of age, usually in the rectum and sigmoid colon. As many as 20% of patients who are affected by bowel cancer may have a family history. Around 10% of colorectal cancers may be caused by a genetic susceptibility. In particular, the Ashkenazi Jewish population has an increased risk of developing bowel cancer, and 5% of this population may carry an altered APC gene, which predisposes to colorectal cancer.

High-risk groups

Familial adenomatous polyposis (FAP)

This condition arises from germ-line alterations in the APC gene on chromosome 5q21-22, and accounts for 1% of patients affected with colorectal cancer. Affected cases may develop hundreds of adenomas by the second to third decade of life, which invariably give rise to colorectal cancer if prophylactic colectomy is not performed. This is performed early, and is followed by annual sigmoidoscopy of the residual rectal area. There are extracolonic associations, which include gastric cancers and osteomas. There are also attenuated forms of FAP.

Hereditary non-polyposis colon cancer (HNPCC)

Case 7

A 35-year-old man is worried about his family history. His father was diagnosed with bowel cancer at 43 years of age. He had a paternal uncle who died of a bladder cancer at the age of 55 years, and a paternal grandmother who was diagnosed with endometrial cancer at 60 years of age.

The GP asks herself the following questions. Are these cancers related or are they independent of each other? What is the risk to this man? What, if any, surveillance or screening modalities are available?

HNPCC is an autosomal dominant inherited condition that predisposes to colorectal cancer, and accounts for 5% of hereditary colorectal cancer. The prevalence is around 1 in 500. A mismatch in DNA repair – a defect in the recognition and repair of DNA replication – occurs when there are alterations in so-called mismatch repair genes. In the case of HNPCC, such important genes include MLH1, MSH2 and MSH6.

Microsatellite instability is a marker for HNPCC. Microsatellites are short DNA sequences in which single nucleotides are repeated. During DNA replication, alterations in microsatellites can result in instability, causing either shortened or lengthened areas of repetitive sequences. The role of mismatch repair proteins is to repair this instability. Thus when microsatellites affect the coding regions, there may be altered protein function. Immunohistochemistry can be used to determine protein expression of mismatch repair genes in tumour tissue. If staining of the relevant proteins is weak or absent, this can indicate which of the mismatch repair genes may be altered.

Colonic tumours in HNPCC tend to predominate on the right side of the colon. There is also an association with other tumour types, including endometrial cancers, gastric cancers and urothelial cancers.

Making a diagnosis

The clinical diagnosis of HNPCC can be made using the so-called Amsterdam criteria. Families can be classed as HNPCC families even if they do not meet the Amsterdam criteria (which were originally used for research studies). People who meet these criteria have a five times higher relative risk of dying from colorectal cancer. The important aspect to consider here is the verification of tumour types, which will help to determine whether these families are in fact HNPCC families.

Box 5.3 The Amsterdam criteria

- Three relatives on the same side of the family with either colorectal cancer or an HNPCC-related cancer, such as endometrial, gastric, small bowel or urothelial cancer.
- One relative should be a first-degree relative of the other two.
- At least two successive generations must be affected.
- At least one cancer must be diagnosed before 50 years of age.
- Familial adenomatous polyposis must be excluded.
- Tumours must be verified by histological examinations/reports.

Patients who fulfil the criteria (such as Case 7 above) should be referred for genetic counselling with a view to genetic testing for the mismatch repair genes. The principle is to initially test a family member who has already developed colorectal cancer or an HNPCC-associated cancer. Cascade testing of other family members at risk could then follow if an identifiable altered mismatch gene is identified.

Surveillance of FAP and high-risk HNPCC

Affected individuals who are carrying an altered APC gene require regular sigmoidoscopy, starting in adolescence, and because of the high risk of upper gastrointestinal malignancy they also require upper gastrointestinal endoscopy examination of the stomach and duodenum. Genetic testing for the APC gene is important in kindred of affected family members. FAP is one genetic condition in which genetic testing is done under the age of 18 years, to look for the altered APC gene.

In those who are already affected with an HNPCC-type cancer, or who are at high risk of developing this type of cancer (50%), colonoscopy every 2 years from the age of 25 years is recommended. As colorectal cancers in HNPCC occur on the right side of the colon, it is vital to ensure that the operator is proficient in reaching the terminal ileum. Small studies of HNPCC families have indicated that colonoscopy surveillance can lead to a 65% reduction in overall mortality.

When considering extracolonic tumours associated with HNPCC, it is not really possible to offer disease surveillance which has proven benefit in reducing mortality. The important principle is to educate patients about their risks and warn them about suspicious symptoms.

Low- to moderate-risk groups

Positive family histories

If the family history does not indicate a high-risk family then depending on the number of affected family members and the age at presentation, it is possible to develop a risk assessment strategy and thus a management plan with regard to surveillance. Case–control studies have indicated the lifetime risk and the relative odds ratio of dying from colorectal cancer.

Consider the next three family pedigrees and determine whether they might be low, moderate or high risk.

Case 8

A 35-year-old man with a 75-year-old father diagnosed with colorectal cancer and a 69-year-old uncle who died of leukaemia.

Case 9

A 29-year-old woman whose mother had colorectal cancer at the age of 43 years.

Case 10

A 44-year-old man whose mother was diagnosed with colorectal cancer at 62 years of age and whose sister was diagnosed with the same cancer at 54 years of age.

Epidemiological case–control studies, prospective cohort studies and life tables to estimate risk have shown that there is an increased relative risk, based on family pedigrees, of developing colorectal cancer if an individual has an affected first-degree relative. Clearly, a shared environment and this interaction between environment and genetics may lead to an increased lifetime risk of developing bowel cancer in the absence of a strongly dominant gene disorder.

The two clinical factors that correlate with an increased familial risk are the number of first-degree relatives affected, and the age at cancer diagnosis.

Box 5.4 Risk stratification based on family history (lifetime risk of developing colorectal cancer based on number and degree of family members affected)

Population risk	1 in 25
One first-degree relative	1 in 17
One first- and one second-degree relative	1 in 12
One first-degree relative aged <45 years	1 in 10
Two first-degree relatives	1 in 6

Thus in applying this to our cases:

Case 8: 35-year-old man with a 75-year-old father diagnosed with colorectal cancer and a 69-year-old uncle who died of leukaemia.

This 35-year-old man has around a 1 in 17 lifetime risk of developing colorectal cancer. His risk is such that he does not need surveillance other than general population screening.

Case 9: 29-year-old woman whose mother had colorectal cancer at the age of 43 years.

This woman's risk is around 1 in 10. With one first-degree relative affected under the age of 45 years, a colonoscopy at the ages of 35 and 55 years would be recommended.[7] She has a moderate risk of developing colon cancer.

Case 10: 44-year-old man whose mother was diagnosed with colorectal cancer at 62 years of age and whose sister was diagnosed with the same cancer at 54 years of age.

With two first-degree relatives affected and the average age less than 60 years, the risk is likely to be less than 1 in 10 and as high as 1 in 6. This man is at moderately high risk, and warrants colonoscopy every 5 years from the age of 45 years, or 5 years before the age of the earliest onset of colon cancer, whichever is latest.

Screening and surveillance

Screening is recommended for those family members who have a lifetime risk of 1 in 10 or higher, which includes those with one affected first-degree relative under the age of 45 years, or two affected first-degree relatives.[7] These people should be assessed and advised by a genetics service to exclude an autosomal dominant condition such as HNPCC.

Screening is recommended at around the age of 35 years and again at 55 years of age by colonoscopy. Clearly, if adenomatous polyps are found, closer surveillance will be needed.

Screening recommendations must include a discussion of the risks and benefits of undergoing colonoscopy, including the risk of perforation.

Those individuals whose risk, based on their family history, is around the general population risk or slightly higher than this should be warned about bowel symptoms and placed on any available national screening programme.

To conclude this section, consider a variation on the first HNPCC case.

Case 7 variation

A 35-year-old man is worried about his family history. His father was diagnosed with bowel cancer at 43 years of age, he had a paternal uncle who died of a bladder cancer at the age of 55 years, and he had a paternal grandmother who was diagnosed with endometrial cancer at 60 years of age. He is unaware, as his mother never told him, that his father with the adverse family history is his parent, but not his biological father. His mother is still living, and has knowledge of his concerns.

This type of case is likely to be more common than was first thought. In essence, the patient believes that he has an adverse family history that may require intrusive investigation or surveillance. But in fact he has no such genetic risk, as his paternal genetic contribution lies elsewhere.

Presumably his mother can reliably attribute his paternity to another individual, although of course this might not be so. If she had had (at least) two sexual partners around the time of this patient's conception, even this aspect would be uncertain. What, if anything, should be done? It can be assumed that our patient's GP knows nothing about the problem, although there are situations where genetic investigation can reveal this 'unplanned' knowledge to the health care professionals alone.[8]

It is tempting to argue that this patient's mother should, at this juncture, reveal his true paternity. Such an argument could be based on his right to know his genetic origin, or on the fact that his best interests would not be served by repeating lower gastrointestinal investigations to no effect.

Against this could be mounted a utilitarian argument that the outcome of this patient's mother revealing her doubts about his paternity could be incendiary – the family might become permanently split. Readers will no doubt have their own perspectives on the correct course of action for the mother. Also of concern is the possibility that this patient will endure inappropriate investigation, not just because it is against his best interests, but also because it constitutes a waste of scarce genetic resources.

Summary

This chapter has reviewed the more common genetically related cancer conditions, and has summarised the statistical risks involved. The role of primary care in assessing the impact of the family history has been considered, and it is suggested that these risks can be more fully evaluated and counselled in that setting.

References

1. Westwood G *et al.* Feasibility and acceptability of providing nurse counsellor genetics clinics in primary care. *J Adv Nurs.* 2006; **53:** 591–604.

2. Emery J, Walton R, Murphy M *et al.* Computer support for interpreting family histories of breast and ovarian cancer in primary care: comparative study with simulated cases. *BMJ.* 2000; **321:** 28–32.

3. The Breast Cancer Consortium. Cancer risks in BRCA2 mutation carriers. *J Natl Cancer Inst.* 1999; **91:** 1310–16.

4. National Institute for Clinical Excellence (NICE). *Familial Breast Cancer. The classification and care of women at risk of familial breast cancer in primary, secondary and tertiary care.* NICE Clinical Guideline 41, developed by the National Collaborating Centre for Primary Care. London: NICE; 2006.

5. For an easy-to-read summary of UKFOCSS, see www.breakthrough.org.uk/about_breast_cancer/family_history/research_and_trials/clinical_trials/uk_familial.html (accessed 13 March 2007).

6. Houlston RS *et al.* Screening and genetic counselling for relatives of patients with colorectal cancer in a family cancer clinic. *BMJ.* 1990; **301:** 366–8.

7. Dunlop MG. Guidance on large bowel surveillance for people with two first-degree relatives with colorectal cancer or one first-degree relative diagnosed with colorectal cancer under 45 years. *Gut.* 2002; **51 (Suppl. V):** v17–20.

8. Parker M, Lucassen A. Concern for families and individuals in clinical genetics. *J Med Ethics.* 2003; **29:** 70–73.

6

Ethical dilemmas and legal cases in primary care genetics

Introduction

This chapter will examine in some detail the main issues in ethics and genetics that have not been covered elsewhere in the book. Three areas of particular interest have been selected. Each of these areas have a particular resonance for primary care, and afford an opportunity for a detailed ethical analysis, particularly with reference to some useful theoretical approaches.

Confidentiality: the moral structure

As has already been stated, the subject of genetic care generates much ethical debate, and perhaps the most challenging theme is that of the clinical duty of confidentiality between health care professional and patient.

Firstly, let us review why there is indeed such a duty of confidence. In ethical terms, four justifications are generally cited.

- It is a duty first described by Hippocrates, who tellingly suggested that our 'secrets should not be noised abroad.'[1] Since then, doctors have been instructed to keep their patients' secrets. In ancient Greek times, Hippocrates related the duty as part of the character or virtue of his learners. It is therefore consistent with the foundations of European moral philosophy.
- Later philosophers, such as Immanuel Kant, developed a more formal theory of duties. When we now describe a *duty* of confidence, we lean heavily on Kant's work.[2]
- We can also argue that if there were no duty of confidentiality, patients would not share their stories with clinicians, and thus it would be impossible to provide care. This aspect highlights another moral theory, known as consequentialism, which accords moral value to those actions that bring about the best outcome.[3]
- A conception of rights, springing from English, French and American roots, offers a last explanation for the duty of confidence, where patients might claim a right to privacy with regard to their clinical information.

Several points need to be added to this necessarily brief summary of moral theory.

It is overtly a summary of European and American thinking on the issues of confidentiality. In Islamic or Chinese ethics, for example, the duty of confidence is less accepted, and therefore breaches of the duty (justified or otherwise) are more easily accommodated. Different cultures and societies may make *relativist* decisions about confidentiality – decisions that are *relatively* different but morally appropriate for that culture or society. In the field of genetics, this area is undeveloped.

Genetic decisions that are made by clinicians touch on all four of these moral theories. For example, the theory of consequentialism would hold that what is morally correct is defined by the best outcome. Therefore a breach of the duty of confidence is entirely moral if the consequences for all are better than they would otherwise have been. A key aspect of consequentialism is that it is the outcomes for all that are relevant, not just those for the patient whose confidence has been breached.

Consider the following case:

Case study

E consults his general practitioner after developing headaches, and he is found to have hypertension. The GP runs the usual work-up of investigations for the newly diagnosed patient, and E returns to the practice nurse for follow-up. She notes that E has been found to have a markedly high total cholesterol level, and a lipid ratio that, according to guidelines, requires treatment. E is happy to consent to treatment with a statin as part of his further management.

In conversation, it emerges that E's son is also a patient of the practice. As a first-degree relative, he is at risk of inheriting his parent's hyperlipidaemia. The nurse suggests to E that she should contact E's son to discuss his situation further and offer further care. E refuses to permit this, as he does not want his family to worry about his own condition, and he therefore prefers to keep the results of his work-up private.

Primary care clinicians will easily recognise this type of conversation. Sharing the care of family members is one of the key features of primary care, and therefore conflicts in the duty of confidence are a common occurrence.

Breaches in the duty of confidentiality

So we now move on to the second aspect of the duty of confidence – where there may be justifications for a breach of it.

Under consequentialist theory, the nurse would be quite right to ignore E's preferences, contact his son and invite him in for investigation, as such an action could uncover a treatable health risk and prevent serious illness. Here the outcome does not concern E alone, but all the people who might be affected by E claiming a right to privacy over information about his own health. This right to privacy would inevitably be undermined if the nurse did speak to his son.

The first justification has been briefly described above, but in fact underlies all common practical applications. From consequentialism, we may say that where there is a harm, or potential harm, to a particular person or persons, then there is a justification for a breach of the duty of confidence. In a non-genetic scenario, this type of breach occurs when one patient suffers from a serious transmissible disease, such as hepatitis B or HIV/AIDS, thus putting a sexual partner at risk.

Equally, if an index patient might transmit an infectious disease to the community, there is a justification for a clinician breaching the patient's confidence to a public health authority that can implement the appropriate disease control measures. These latter actions are both ethically justified within consequentialism, and this justification also lies behind the public health law that can be used to prevent disease spread. The precise details of public health law will vary between countries, although they will retain the same ethical roots. Clearly, this consequentialist justification is at odds with a strict interpretation of the duty of confidentiality, and is certainly at odds with the right to privacy, as E claims above.

The second justification for a breach of a duty of confidence is easier to comprehend, and simply relies on an autonomous decision by a patient. For instance, if E can be encouraged by the clinical team to allow information about his lipid status to be shared with his son, then a frank discussion can be held. E would be consenting to the breach of a duty of confidentiality, and it would therefore be ethically correct. It is a feature of the sharing of genetic information that E's son will have to know of its origin in E's work-up, and the hereditable nature of the problem.

The key issue here is that information about hereditary illnesses is relevant to all family members. However, decision making about the sharing of such information can be very difficult, regardless of how it comes to light. In the above example, E has limited the degree to which his diagnosis may be shared, but is he right to do that?

Let us now consider whether E's son might argue that he has a right to know about a familial illness. He could argue that it is impossible for him to make full decisions about his life unless he knows about his cardiac risk factors, for example, including his cholesterol level. That would not preclude him from seeking health advice from the practice in his own right, independent of his father's actions.

In all likelihood, E's diagnosis of hyperlipidaemia would come as a surprise to him, and might spark off consideration of his own health status. Neither of these observations do much to advance the idea that E's son could claim a right to such knowledge.

Rights and privacy

Rights theory teaches us that for every right there must be a *correlative* duty such that the holder of the right can demand the implementation of the right by another who must have such a duty to give it. For example, if it is agreed that E's son has a right to the lipid information, then someone else, either E himself or his clinicians, must have a duty to provide it. The nature of the duties would be family or professionally based, respectively.[4]

The rights argument is more plausibly argued from a position that family health information, like other types of information within families, is intrinsically shared – it cannot be anything else. All that health care professionals do is to bring it to light under a duty of care. When that is so, it should be freely available to the family so that they can make their own decisions about what to do in the circumstances.

Given a right as described, there is a correlative duty on E to reveal the information to his son and others. Might there be a duty for someone else to reveal this information to E's son if E will not do so? Alternatively, put another way, what is the scope of the team's professional duty to E's son?

A different kind of argument seems to operate here. If E's son were not a patient of the practice, there would be no professional or legal duty, but there might still be a moral duty. As he is a patient of the practice, there may be a professional duty to inform him because there is a pre-existent duty of care. To try to resolve this aspect of the problem, consider some variations. Hyperlipidaemia is part of a multifactorial genesis of cardiovascular disease, and is at least partially treatable by diet or drugs. We might say, therefore, that it is a potentially serious problem and that it is modifiable. Consider, assuming that a duty to inform E's son is a given, whether the same would apply if the disease in question was either more or less serious.

It could be argued that if the disease that the general practitioner identified in E was, say, Gilbert's syndrome,[5] and therefore of less consequence to his son, the team would not be under a duty to breach their duty of confidence to E and inform his son. In other words, the gravity of the disorder defines the duty to disclose, and perhaps also the right of E's son to be given the information.

On the other hand, if the nature of the disorder was more serious than hyperlipidaemia, then we might say that there is even more need to disclose its nature to E's son. If the disorder that was discovered was a hereditary neuromuscular disease such as myotonic dystrophy, relatively resistant to treatment, then perhaps not only E's son but also other members of the family should be entitled to know, and the practice team might be the only agency of their knowing.

However, in such a situation, it has been said that there is a right 'not to know', as the disease is not treatable, and if family members are told, they will have several additional years of anxiety before the onset of the disease itself.[6] These arguments have been examined at length in the case of family members of sufferers of Huntington's disease. Readers will know that this is a particularly devastating condition, in which dementia and neurological disease appear in adult life, and that it is associated with a dominant-gene mode of transmission. If the disease is diagnosed in an individual, then family members are at risk and can be offered appropriate testing which, if positive, in most cases defines future disease progress. The question thus arises, as with E, as to whether relatives who may be at risk should be warned of this. Huntington's disease is unarguably serious, and identifiable in those at risk.

Even though we might attach great importance to autonomous decision making as representative of its pre-eminence as a principle for the index case, E's family have their own autonomous decisions to make, too, and illnesses such as Huntington's disease have the capacity to undermine autonomous decision making like no others. What can be posited here is a conflict between a 'duty to warn' on the part of the clinical team and a 'right to know' on the part of the family members.

Disclosure and the law

Courts in the USA have begun deciding to uphold the 'right to know' about adverse genetic information,[7] thus requiring clinicians to disclose to family members their risk. In doing so, these courts are interpreting and applying a longstanding decision (the case of *Tarasoff*[8]). Here a duty to disclose was developed from a situation where a person known to be at risk of harm from a violent criminal was eventually killed by him. The murderer had shared his thoughts with a counsellor who, it was held, had not warned the police of the potential harm adequately enough for the murder to be prevented. Thus, in the USA, the risk of serious harm to an individual obliges the clinician to breach confidentiality if that harm might be prevented.

Tarasoff is not binding in other jurisdictions, so a duty to warn is not part of the law outside the USA. In any event, the fact that the law is binding in one jurisdiction does not make it morally binding in another. Furthermore, it could be said that the existence of a law that requires a breach of confidence is not the same thing as rendering that law morally correct.

The leading British case on this issue agreed that a clinician could breach a duty of confidence to prevent serious harm, but did not establish a duty in law to do so. In this case, a prisoner who was serving a long term tried to bring an action against a psychiatrist, for disclosing to the authorities his report that the prisoner was potentially dangerous. Again, because of the risk of violence, the court held that a breach of confidence and a disclosure were lawful, but did not go so far as to say that it was necessarily a duty on the doctor to disclose.[8]

UK law is also concerned with statutes or Acts of Parliament – those parts of the law enacted by legislative process. In the area of clinical confidentiality, the relevant statute is the *Data Protection Act 1998*. This law covers many areas that are relevant to health care professionals, detailing their responsibilities when handling personal information, and the rights of the patient (or *data subject*, in the jargon). In fact this law was the result of incorporating a European Data Protection Directive into UK law. The law contains no particular content on genetic information, as it is mainly concerned with individual consent to, among other things, retention and handling of personal information. There has been academic discussion about the scope of the law, including the observation that even holding a family history could be unlawful, as the consent of the individuals in the family, who have been alluded to by the index patient, has not been obtained.

In summary, it has been difficult to substantiate the claim that there is a legal 'duty to disclose', on the part of the health care professional who has a duty of care, beyond the index genetic case. Nonetheless, whatever the law may say in all its formality, the moral terrain needs to be considered, as it is more useful to the clinician wrestling with dilemmas such as those in the case of E.

Professional guidelines on confidentiality

Clinicians, while recognising the importance of the legal principles already discussed, will also have access to their own profession's guidance, which takes into account relevant law and ethics.

At the outset, the distinction between legal, moral and professional rules should be borne in mind. They clearly overlap, but have different functions. This section will focus on the professional guidelines.

The professional body for all UK doctors is the General Medical Council (GMC), a self-regulating[9] organisation that controls who joins (and leaves) the Medical Register, offers guidance on clinical practice and has sundry other functions. The GMC has issued current guidelines on consent[10] and confidentiality[11] which, taken together, require the following actions of UK doctors.

Consent by the patient to the sharing of information is generally required, but the duty of confidence is not absolute, and there are occasions when it may be breached, as in the examples above.

The GMC guidance was adopted in 2006 by the Joint Committee on Medical Genetics in their statement on the sharing of genetic information.[12] Not surprisingly, they highlight the importance of consent to such sharing, but recognise that there are circumstances in which a non-consensual disclosure of genetic information may take place.

Such circumstances would necessarily include an attempt to persuade the index patient to disclose a genetic illness of such seriousness as to make the disclosure not only outweigh any distress to the patient, but also the clinician discussing the case with senior colleague(s). Readers may wish to reflect on whether the disclosure of E's lipid status to his son falls within these strictures – or indeed whether arguably more serious illnesses, such as Huntington's disease, might do so.

Given the continuing relationships between primary care practitioners and their patients, and the fact of caring for families rather than, necessarily, for individuals, such decisions are likely to be handled more often in primary care in the future.

The Joint Committee acknowledges another category of consent in information-sharing matters, not previously noted. This is where the consent to disclosure is unclear.[13] This may be because of the passage of time, inaccessibility of the index patient or something similar, and is more relevant to consent decisions about the use of samples that have already been provided. Nonetheless, advice is given that disclosure of genetically important facts may be undertaken in these circumstances if it is in the best interests of the family member.

Designed babies and family responsibilities

Altruism and families

Issues inherent in reproduction have been considered in Chapter 3, without acknowledging a newly emerging and related technology. It has been shown with the advent of pre-implantation genetic testing (PIGD) and *in-vitro* fertilisation (IVF) that sperm, ova and fetuses can be assessed for their value to existing children.

The process works like this. If an existing child suffers from a serious illness such as leukaemia or Diamond–Blackfan anaemia, one therapeutic option may be a bone-marrow transplant from a suitable donor. If there is no match in the immediate family, there is the possibility that the parents of the afflicted child could conceive another child with the express purpose of making that second child a donor. PIGD and IVF can ensure that the second child's tissues match.

Two subsidiary points need to be made at the outset. First, it is unlikely that primary care will have much to do with the technical aspects of the delivery of such care. The procedures involved are only performed in secondary care facilities, and are very much at the leading edge of clinical practice. The role of GPs and their teams will be essentially supportive, focusing on the care of the parents and the existing children.

Box 6.1 Diamond–Blackfan anaemia

This rare congenital disorder is characterised by defective erythropoiesis. In early infancy, affected patients may present with a normochromic or macrocytic anaemia, and the disorder is associated with limb, urogenital or cardiovascular malformations. There is also an increased risk of leukaemia. Treatment includes repeated blood transfusions leading to associated long-term complications. Most cases are sporadic. However, in 10% of cases inheritance may occur through a dominant or, less commonly, a recessive pattern. In up to 25% of patients, mutations have been found on chromosome 19q13.2 encoding ribosomal protein S19.

Secondly, donations of human tissue from one family member to another are in themselves actions of moral value. It is the fact that families share genetic material that makes donation possible at all, and the closer a family member is to the affected person, the more likely it is that there will be a tissue match. Should a match occur, it is important to consider the nature of the transaction beyond the technical or clinical. Initially it would seem that a donation to a family member is a freely consensual and altruistic action to the benefit of the index patient. However, it is more complicated than that. For example, the matched donor may feel pressure to donate simply because there is a match. Consider it like this. When families are tested with the aim of helping one of them who has a serious and possibly lethal disease, and only one family member turns out to be a match, it can be difficult to rethink participation without some family dissent.

Of course, no one can be tested for a match with the index patient without their consent, but that consent may change over time, or even in response to finding out that there is a match.

A larger and more theoretical analysis of this area would examine the nature of the responsibility of family members to one another. In other words, it would examine how commonalities of genetics connect with relationships or internal responsibilities. It has been said that the closer the genetic connection, the greater our responsibilities to one another. Therefore such responsibilities would be greatest to first-degree relatives, and least to non-relatives. If this is so, then expectations that close relatives will donate tissue or organs are reasonably high.

Against this notion may be argued the degree of risk inherent in donating tissue. In the case of tissues such as blood, the risk to the donor is vanishingly small. Blood is actually the most commonly donated human tissue. Bone marrow is more complicated to donate. It is more uncomfortable and carries a slightly higher risk than venepuncture, but it is difficult to imagine the risk to the donor outweighing the benefit to the patient with a disease such as leukaemia. However, that very fact might increase pressure on the donor to donate, rendering the quality of their consent less clear. Donation of a solid organ such as a kidney, which involves a surgical procedure of greater complexity, inevitably carries a higher risk of complications. One is justified in asking whether the altruistic decision to assist and probably save the life of a relative is as freely consensual as the decision to consent to a personal clinical intervention.

The UK law in this area is now regulated by the Human Tissue Act 2004,[14] the precise details of which need not concern us here.

Creating babies for a reason

This rather loaded heading conceals the fact that most babies *are* created for a reason – the continuation of the species and the propagation of families, or at least the next generations. Whether those reasons obtain at the time of every act of sexual intercourse is more difficult to say.

The reason under discussion in this section is the best interests and welfare of an existing, seriously ill sibling. In moral terms, what needs to be examined is whether it is right for children to be conceived and selected purposefully for the welfare of their 'siblings to be.'

This possibility has only arisen by virtue of recent advances in genetic and assisted reproduction. It is not a moral dilemma that could have been considered prior to this (an observation that is common to many medical ethical dilemmas).

Several strands are relevant here. One of Kant's most enduring moral 'imperatives' was that individuals should always be ends in themselves and never only means, and he regarded this as being of primary importance. He was suggesting that as humans we cannot serve only as the means to bring about other things, but that we are of value in ourselves.[15] In contrast, animals, being morally irrelevant, may serve the need to satiate our hunger, representing an end. A religious view of this topic might include the descriptor 'sacred.' Thus humans possess some special quality, or sacredness, that gives them an intrinsic value endowed by a creator. If we were to conceive a person with the express aim of serving some other purpose, such as saving a sibling, then worthy as this aim is, it does not conform to the moral criteria stated above.[16]

However, the purposefully conceived fetus will have a value – an instrumental value – by virtue of the benefit that it can confer on its afflicted sibling, in addition to its intrinsic value. There is also the possibility that its particular genetic make-up may have come about by chance alone, rather than by human agency. So one way of looking at this new fetus is that the odds of genetic shuffling that occur at the time of fertilisation and before have simply been loaded by high-technology intervention.

Given that the germ cells, fetus and child in that order are the subjects of the decision, there can be no notion of consent to the whole process. Any consent must emanate from the parents, who would have the best interests of the afflicted child at heart. Indeed they would not have initiated the treatment if this were not so.

From a utilitarian viewpoint, so long as the risks to the new fetus are minimal, there would seem to be no moral problem. On the positive side, a child may be saved by the donation of tissue from the sibling created, or at the very least selected, for that purpose. On the negative side would weigh the risks to all concerned. Side-effects might include the commodification of persons so created.

These issues have been examined in a legal case in the UK, where the parents of a child with β-thalassaemia disease sought leave from the courts[17] to create a new sibling selected to be suitable as a tissue donor. The nature of the putative donation was retention of cord blood with its stem-cell content at the time of delivery. The origin of the case was a challenge by a pressure group to the legality of the Human Fertilisation and Embryology Authority[18] in agreeing to the process. The facts of the case help us to reach a moral judgement on this and similar cases.

First, the mother of the affected child had three other normal children, older than the affected boy, who did not provide a tissue match. She had had two further pregnancies – one was another β-thalassaemia major fetus who was aborted, and another did not match. Clearly, the parents had tried to load the odds to help their son, without success.

Secondly, it was not at all clear that the UK law permitted the selection of an embryo, after PIGD, tissue typing for HLA and assisted conception, to provide a tissue donor for the afflicted child. In the end, the case turned on whether the HFEA could lawfully allow a 'suitable' embryo to be selected. In eventually allowing that it could, the court declined to comment on whether in other circumstances a 'suitable' embryo could be selected for gender. Strictly, what the court allowed was that the HFEA could license the process.

Thirdly, in doing so the court took note of the nature of the reason for the process, namely that it was directed towards improving the health of the existing child, rather than being due to any other motivation.

In summary, what the court did was to approve a utilitarian move to bring about the creation of one type of person – a specific type – to help another person who needed it. Clearly, this was not something of which Kant would have approved.

The larger issues, which were debated in the professional and lay press at the time, included the possible commodification of children in this way – that is, the notion that unborn children could be viewed as a commodity, a package of DNA useful to a third party. Other issues included the difficulty of establishing the best interests of the existing child should the procedure fail, and the societal attitudes to the process.[19]

The problem of personal insurance

The issue of access to life insurance is relevant to anyone who seeks to take out a mortgage, or who requires life insurance for other financial reasons. Life insurance premiums are largely dependent on health status. Insurers are generally not keen to insure people with lower than average life expectancy, as the financial risk is greater. The system that they operate is a risk pool based on the principle of mutuality. A company's customers pool their risk of death or serious illness, and over time, enough people survive and pay their contributions to generate profit for the company. High-risk individuals may be excluded from cover, so that they do not prejudice the risk pool too much and lead to excessive financial risk to the company.

Similarly, the UK National Health Service is a risk pool, although the population does not pay at the time of use. Patients at high or low risk of illness draw their benefit as health care according to need. No differentiation is made for those at high risk, and the principle applied is known as *solidarity*.

There is a particular issue in genetic disease, as a particular genetic make-up may be associated with future disease – in much the same way as a known attribute such as hypercholesterolaemia may be associated with future disease. In addition, a documented family history can attribute genetic risk of disease to another person. This is conceivably of great interest to insurance companies, who may reduce their financial risk by excluding individuals with genetic markers of disease, in the same way that exclusions are made now for active life-limiting conditions.

Primary care doctors in particular hold long-term records on patients, more so than other health care providers, and those records may include family history records, genetic test records and other markers of disease. Such information is of relevance in assessing insurance risk, and it is sought and provided by general practitioners, provided that patient consent is sought and given. At least in the UK, GPs are more used to working within the principle of solidarity – that is, not excluding individuals at high risk from access to care. By releasing personal information, GPs become involved with the insurance principle of mutuality, with which they are not generally so familiar.

In fact, insurers and patients have agreed that there should be restrictions on the transfer and use of genetic information when determining personal health risk for insurance purposes. This agreement is known as the *Concordat and Moratorium on Genetics and Insurance*, and it was implemented in the UK on 1 November 2006 for 5 years, including a review in 2008. In fact this agreement extends a prior arrangement on a similar basis.[20] The *Concordat* is an interesting document for all sorts of reasons, but the items of interest to primary care doctors are summarised below.

- Customers (patients) will not be pressured to undergo predictive genetic testing.
- Customers will not be asked to disclose relatives' genetic test results.
- Insurers may seek customers' family history and diagnostic genetic test results from customers themselves or their GPs, with consent.
- Insurers may ask customers to disclose predictive adverse genetic test results where policies exceed £500,000 for life policies (or £300,000 for critical illness policies, and £30,000 for income protection policies).
- Insurers will not treat those customers who have adverse predictive test results less favourably without justification.
- The use of predictive genetic tests will remain under consideration and be subject to oversight.

Some of this material calls for expansion. The term *diagnostic* in this context means confirmation of a diagnosis of ill health (e.g. where a haemoglobinopathy is identified). The term *predictive* is used to denote a marker of future disease, and the agreement is mainly concerned with disorders that can be foreseen. An example would be a gene marker for IHD or diabetes as described in the section above.

Being an agreement, the *Concordat* is not law, or even quasi-law,[21] but a non-binding arrangement between relevant parties to constrain an otherwise quite normal business practice, namely the assessment of financial risk. Only 97% of insurance companies in the UK are members of the Association of British Insurers, which slightly limits its observance.

There is also an intriguing clause allowing the insurers to apply for the use of predictive tests for monogenic, late-onset or high-penetrance disorders. This could be regarded as an 'escape clause', permitting the use of such tests to identify patients at high risk who could then be excluded from cover.

If a patient has a high-risk history, they are often required to undergo biochemical tests before cover is commenced. A high-risk history might include excessive alcohol consumption, or indeed an identified hyperlipidaemia as in E's case. If insurers were successful in applying for predictive tests under the *Concordat,* these tests would be performed and risk calculations would be adjusted.

There is a view that insurers do not need access to genetic testing of this kind in order to calculate risk of future disease, and that all that is needed is a family history of the potential customer. One insurer opted out of an earlier form of the *Concordat* for that reason.[22] Customers are asked to disclose known family patterns of illness, and it has been said that familial breast cancer, colon cancer, Huntington's disease and adult polycystic renal disease cover most of the financially significant diagnoses. Thus if an insurer adjusts a premium in line with actuarial predictions for mortality for these conditions, a predictive test is unlikely to add very much to their financial calculation, or the client's premium.[23]

The dilemma for the GP concerns the release of information about family history when the customer (or patient) has consented to the submission of a personal medical report to the potential insurer. Given the discussion about confidentiality in the first section of this chapter, respect for the principle of autonomy would suggest that the consent renders the release ethical.

However, there are three areas which might give the GP cause for concern here. First, it is information about a third party to the transaction – that is, the relative who is him- or herself the owner of the family history. Normally no consent is sought or taken from this relative, but it is their personal history that affects the financial decision. Secondly, the information about the family is disclosed, presumably, by the patient at the time of registration, or it might come with old records from previous GPs and others. This feature is peculiar to the UK and other health systems that operate a universal and registerable relationship with individuals. Just as information that primary care teams hold about patients is to some extent challengeable, information about their relatives must be considered more so.

Thirdly, when a GP provides a report to an insurer about a patient (or customer), there is a double duty in operation – one to the patient and another to the insurer. Sometimes this is a complicated set of duties if they can be held to be in opposition. If the GP's report about a family history leads to the refusal, deferment or loading of a policy, it can hardly be said to be in the best interests of the patient.

Summary

This chapter has examined some of the key ethico-legal issues in primary care genetics, not dealt with elsewhere in this book. It is clear that the relationship between ethics and law in this field is not always straightforward, and that the law does not have the answers to all of the moral dilemmas that arise. As such, genetics is like any other field. Where it differs is in the presence of third parties and the complexities that they cause for clinicians and patients alike.

References

1. Many translations of the Hippocratic Oath exist, with slight English variations. This version is from the University of Adelaide; http://etext.library.adelaide.edu.au/h/hippocrates/h7w/oath.html (accessed 3 March 2007).

2. Rachels J. *Elements of Moral Philosophy*. 5th ed. McGraw-Hill Higher Education; 2006. This provides a good introduction to the work of Immanuel Kant.

3. Brief descriptions of consequentialism and rights are to be found in Boyd KM, Higgs R, Pinching AJ, editors. *The New Dictionary of Medical Ethics*. London: BMJ Publications; 1997. More detailed analysis of these moral theories can be found in Beauchamp T, Childress J. *Principles of Biomedical Ethics*. Oxford: Oxford University Press; 2001.

4. Leung Wai-Ching *et al.* Results of genetic testing: when confidentiality conflicts with a duty to warn relatives. *BMJ*. 2002; **321:** 1464–9. Here several authors analyse a similar case, with one describing the nature of a putative family duty.

5. See Chapter 4 for an account of Gilbert's syndrome.

6. Wilcke J. Late-onset genetic disease: where ignorance is bliss, is it folly to inform relatives? *BMJ*. 1998; **317:** 744–7. This is a cogent article describing similar problems in the case of a-1-antitrypsin deficiency.

7. Offit K, Groeger E, Turner S *et al.* The 'duty to warn' a patient's family members about hereditary disease risks. *JAMA*. 2004; **292:** 1469–73. This article provides a full review of the cases.

8. The full reports can be found in *W v Egdell 1990 Ch 359* [1990] 1 All ER 835, but a good discussion can be found in *Law and Medical Ethics*. 7th ed. Mason JK and Laurie GT, OUP; 2005, ISBN 978-0199282395.

9. Self-regulation is a longstanding aspect of statutory medical organisation in the UK. This is correct at the time of writing, but may not remain quite so true in the light of recent recommendations. The latest UK Government proposals are revealed in the following White Paper: Department of Health. *Trust, Assurance and Safety: the regulation of health professionals*. London: Department of Health; 2007.

10. General Medical Council. *Seeking Patients' Consent: the ethical considerations*. London: General Medical Council; 1998.

11. General Medical Council. *Confidentiality: protecting and providing information*. London: General Medical Council; 2004.

12. Farndon P, Douglas F, editors. *Consent and Confidentiality in Genetic Practice: guidance on genetic testing and sharing genetic information*. London: Joint Committee on Medical Genetics of the Royal College of Physicians, the Royal College of Pathologists and the British Society for Human Genetics; 2006.

13. Ibid., para 2.5.2.

14. The full text of this new statute can be found at www.hmso.gov.uk/acts2004/20040030.htm (accessed 21 December 2007).

15. Ibid.

16. Dworkin R. *Life's Dominion: an argument about abortion, euthanasia and individual freedom.* London: Vintage; 1993. This unsurpassed text provides a full discussion of the sacredness and intrinsic value of life. Extracts from it can be found in Dworkin R. What is sacred? In: Harris J, editor. *Bioethics.* Oxford: Oxford University Press; 2001.

17. *Quintavalle (on behalf of Comment on Reproductive Ethics) v HFEA* [2005] UKHL 28.

18. See Chapter 3 for a full description of the HFEA and its role.

19. Boyle RJ, Savulescu J. Ethics of using pre-implantation genetic diagnosis to select the stem-cell donor for an existing person. *BMJ.* 2001; **323:** 1240–3. This article provides a good expansion of the ethical issues.

20. Department of Health. *Concordat and Moratorium on Genetics and Insurance.* London: Department of Health; 2005. This was agreed between the Association of British Insurers, the Human Genetics Commission, the Genetics and Insurance Commission and the UK Government.

21. Quasi-law can be best understood by reference to professional guidelines issued by bodies such as the General Medical Council (GMC) and the Nursing and Midwifery Council (NMC). These professional guidelines are not strictly legally binding, but would be strongly respected during any legal process. Professionals cannot practise in the UK outwith the GMC or NMC rules.

22. Lenaghan J. In: *A Brave New NHS? The impact of the new genetics on the health service.* London: Institute for Public Policy Research; 1998, ISBN 1860300650. This is a very accessible review of many organisational issues in the field.

23. Ibid.

7

Genetics, genomics and society

Introduction

This chapter will explore some of the challenging issues surrounding clinical care, with particular reference to genomics. The latter issue, of which mention has already been made, is of course one of the most important in the field. Our genomes are our genetic make-up – now potentially identifiable down to the last nucleotide base pair. When we know what our genomes are, and the effect that they can have on ourselves and our illnesses, our lives may change in very many different ways. Some of those changes will be examined below.

Genetics and society

Genetics and legal process

One of the effects of having individual genetic profiles is that the individual with the profile can be traced, followed or associated with events that leave a genetic marker. Put differently, anywhere that we leave our DNA can betray where we have been. In recent years, criminal investigation has been revolutionised by this technology – individuals have been convicted of rape simply by associating DNA found on a victim with DNA in a suspect. This ability hinges on the singularity of a person's DNA make-up.

As a consequence of this kind of technology, a database of DNA profiles is being built up in the UK and elsewhere. It is estimated that 5% of all adults in the UK now have their DNA profile held on this database, and the figure is growing all the time. The implications for criminal investigation are obvious – where a DNA sample is recoverable at a crime scene, the police may be able to recall a profile that gives an immediate match to a suspect on the database.

However, this area is fraught with argument. What should be the entry criteria for the database? To what extent should health care professionals involve themselves in the collection of samples?[1]

There are UK government policies that address these areas.[2] They tend to argue that the larger the database, the better the rate of detection of crime, although these arguments have not gone unchallenged.[3]

Primary care professionals are unlikely to be involved directly in the forensic investigation of crime, but may be approached by other legal authorities to take samples of tissue in order to confirm family relationships. These are now generally buccal scrape specimens, rather than the blood tests that were previously required. The drivers for these investigations emerge from contested paternity or child protection procedures. In cases where court-ordered paternity confirmation tests are required, health care professionals are not in a position to refuse to participate.

If the paternity testing is requested by patients, or more usually by their parents, it is very important to establish that it is actually in the best interests of the child that such testing should proceed. This requires careful consideration of what those interests may mean, and how they might be served by the confirmation, or otherwise, of biological parentage.[4] For example, will the determination result in concrete benefits to the child? Do those benefits depend on the age of the child involved? Will the child be able to contribute to the decision at all?

Health care professionals will no doubt want to add up all the factors before participating in such a process.

Over-the-counter testing

This issue is analogous to others in health care currently in the public domain. Should there be direct advertising of prescription medicines to the public? How much access should individuals have directly to specialists or allied health care professionals? Similarly, should people have direct access to genetic tests on an 'over-the-counter' basis? Precisely which counter is not particularly important, although pharmacies' counters, for obvious reasons, are often quoted.

One of the roles of health care professionals is the translation of their esoteric language into everyday vernacular. In that sense the skill of communication, already referred to in this book in the context of communication of genetic risk, is of great importance. If the public were to have direct access to genetic testing, then inevitably those interpretive skills would be of considerable use.

Some pathology tests are already available in the UK (e.g. pregnancy testing kits. ovulation detection kits). It has been argued that genetic tests are significantly different in their complexity, their interpretability and their impact on individuals other than those tested.[5] Although we would not disagree with the last point, the idea that 'ordinary' tests are simple and easy to discuss with patients is not necessarily true. For example, consider the complexities of interpreting the significance of a blood lipids test, or even a blood pressure result.

In any event, 'over-the-counter' genetic testing is not currently available in the UK, and this position is supported (with one important qualification that will be dealt with below) by the Human Genetics Commission (HGC).[6]

Such testing is available in other parts of the world. For example, in the USA, commercial companies will process ordinary buccal cell samples (taken by simple mouth swabbing) and produce a genetic profile of risk for certain diseases, particularly ischaemic heart disease. This is claimed to be done by genomic analysis, and is described as the new science of *nutrigenomics*. Given the uncertainty of the results in defining (as yet) real risk, and the difficulty of interpreting risk even without unconfirmed genetic testing, such tests cannot be recommended as being necessarily in patients' best interests. Also available in the USA are over-the-counter tests for carrier status (e.g. for thalassaemia or sickle-cell trait).

The qualification referred to above is important for primary care. The UK HGC does not proscribe all such 'over-the-counter' tests, but suggests that those which are made available rely on the agency of primary care as a 'genetically literate workforce' to 'manage and allow access.'[7] Although we would argue for the former description, the latter is self-evidently more problematic.[8] It is in the nature of 'over-the-counter' activity to be outside professionals' control, so quite how access is controlled is unclear. As ever, it is likely that the role of the health care professionals is to interpret the results of patients' self-discovered knowledge, requiring these professionals to be 'genetically literate' in those areas.

Genetics at work

A scenario that the primary care professional might encounter is a patient asking for advice as to whether they should undergo a genetic test, at their employer's request, as a condition prior to employment. So far, genetic testing has not been used systematically by employers in the UK. In the USA, a well-publicised case was highlighted in which an employer used genetic testing of a marker that has been associated with hereditary neuropathy (which gives rise to pressure palsies) as a way of predicting whether the employees would be susceptible to carpal tunnel syndrome.[9] The US congress is considering the Genetic Information Non-Discrimination Act of 2005, which aims to protect citizens against unwarranted genetic testing.[10]

This case highlights a number of reasons why an employer may want to consider a genetic test. The first is that an employer may consider that the nature of the job may predispose and expose susceptible people, with a genetic predisposition, to occupational hazards, which in turn may increase the likelihood of their developing an illness or their health being adversely affected. In effect, the employer is screening for any potential disease, and may use an adverse result to look for early signs of disease as a consequence of exposure to occupational hazards.[8] The factors that would counter this reason for testing, apart from the legal and ethical aspects, would be that the predictive test or clinical utility of genetic testing might be very low, that other issues such as environmental factors may be important, and that improving workplace safety procedures and protocols may be more effective. If an employee were to develop a disease (and be known to have a genetic predisposition), proving a causal link between the disease and the occupation may well be a scientific conundrum.

However, there are instances where a genetic test may be required or requested in the interest of public safety. The classic example that is cited is the pilot with a family history of sudden cardiac death syndrome. Clearly, the ethical and legal ramifications need to be considered carefully in the use of predictive genetic testing.

The Human Genetics Commission (HGC) has clearly stated that 'No person shall be unfairly discriminated against on the basis of his or her genetic characteristics.' Clearly, the UK Disability Discrimination Act 1995[11] as well as human rights declarations would support the notion that anyone who is suffering from a genetic condition should not be precluded from obtaining gainful employment.

The key recommendations made by the HGC in 2002[12] include the following:

- a statement on the use of information that an employer may have on an employee relating to a genetic condition; recognition of the fact that an employer may use the information in a number of different ways, including risk assessment in the workplace, workforce planning, and occupational pensions and insurance

- employers must not demand a pre-employment genetic test as a precondition for employment
- the recognition that predictive personal genetic information is not being used systematically in the UK, and that employers should inform the HGC voluntarily if there are any plans to do so
- further consultation with interested parties and groups should take place.

A recent House of Lords debate[13] highlighted the concern that some felt about genetics in the workplace, and it is likely that a Green Paper for consultation will be published with the HGC's recommendations.

Eubionics and euphenics

In Chapter 3 we considered the reproductive issues that are relevant to genetics, with some reference to the challenging ethical dilemmas contained therein. There are additional areas of interest that are essentially societal. The term 'eubionics' was coined by McNally in 2004, to describe a quest for bodily perfection via the genetic or non-genetic route.[14] McNally suggests that 'eugenics' as generally rendered is an unfortunate and effete term used to describe, among other things, the fact of abortion following an adverse genetic diagnosis. It may have the purpose of collectively making a people different to what they were before – a kind of human 'tidying up.' As such, eugenics is vulnerable to the perversions of the process, as practised by the Nazis.

To be eubionic is to seek bodily improvement, or even perfection, in ourselves and our children by whatever route. Thus this theoretical position tends to subvert any notion of genetic exceptionalism (i.e. that there is anything special about genetic information or decision making). This seems to be congruent with the general aims and objectives of primary care in general.

An earlier author adds to the word salad by coining the term 'euphenics', which is generally taken to mean an improvement in phenotype, and thus overlaps with the meaning of eubionics as above.[15] The difference probably takes account of the concept of the genome, which was not fully acknowledged in 1963.

It is the genome, or our knowledge of it, that gives rise to the possibility of euphenic or eubionic change. If we endorse it, as clinicians our motives may change 'from caring for people to fixing them.'[16] This is a very important aspect of clinical practice, taking in the whole of medical ethics in one way or another. In short, the change captured by this rather snappy phrase is one of primary clinical intent. Should clinicians aim to counteract human suffering as their main professional purpose, or should they be partners in a eubionic enterprise of self-improvement? Perhaps the latter is the role of the scientist, or the salesman.

Pharmacogenetics

To clarify the terminology, *pharmacogenetics* is a term that describes the fact that genetic factors can modify drug action, whereas *pharmacogenomics* involves the analysis of DNA, in particular looking for genomic variations that might be used to predict the response to administered drugs, and to predict adverse drug reactions.[17] This personalisation of pharmacology helps to predict the possible outcomes of therapy, particularly in cancer treatment. The variation in the genome that might give rise to varying drug responses may be accounted for by single nucleotide polymorphisms (SNPs). This can be used to make a genetic map of the variation between individuals, helping to predict variations in drug handling and metabolism. The haplotype refers to groups of SNPs on the same gene, and current research is focusing on developing the Hap Map,[18] a haplotype map that will describe patterns of human DNA variation.

Pharmaceutical companies have been developing technology to make diagnostic tools to try to determine these genetic variations. For example, Roche Diagnostics have developed an AmpliChip technology which uses the microarray technique, a powerful tool that can rapidly analyse literally thousands of genes. Their aim is to characterise individuals who may have the genotype for and perhaps need treatment for depression, cancer or leukaemia.

An example of this is the CYP2D6 enzyme, which is part of the cytochrome P450 enzyme system, and is involved in the metabolism of antidepressant drugs. Variation in the CYP2D6 gene has been associated with variation in drug metabolism, with some patients being poor metabolisers and others being ultra-rapid metabolisers of tricyclic antidepressants and antipsychotic drugs.

Important policy documents have aided the debate in describing the ethical and social aspects of pharmacogenetics,[19] as well as its potential uses.[20] There does appear to be a consensus that the scenario of pharmacogenetically personalised drug administration in routine clinical practice may not occur for another two decades. The complexity of the necessary genetic studies and other factors, such as environmental interactions, ethnic differences in drug metabolism, drug interactions and disease (e.g. renal disease) makes for a rich vein of potential research. It also highlights the difficulty involved in translating research into clinical practice.

However, the primary care physician may already have seen examples of situations where drug treatment can be tailored to a knowledge of the individual's genetic make-up. For example, there are women with breast cancer who express a gene for a tumour growth factor receptor called HER2, and when the gene responsible is over-expressed can respond to treatment with trastuzumab (Herceptin). This drug has been shown to reduce 'time to disease progression' in women with breast cancer, and the drug is only prescribed if multiple copies of the gene that expresses HER2 are present.

In patients who require immunosuppression (e.g. in the treatment of inflammatory bowel disease) and might need to be given azathioprine, it is useful to measure thiopurine methyl transferase (TPMT). This is an important enzyme that is necessary for the metabolism of thiopurine drugs. Mutations in the gene that codes for this enzyme can lead to life-threatening bone-marrow suppression after administration of azathioprine.

Classic examples of the way in which genetic variation may affect drug dosing are the cough associated with ACE inhibitors, which has been linked to bradykinin levels, and the fact that individuals with a deficiency of the enzyme glucose-6-phosphate dehydrogenase are at risk of anaemia following the administration of antimalarial drugs.

With regard to the administration of warfarin, anything that reduces the risk of bleeding should be welcomed, but it is clear that further research will be necessary to achieve this. Two common variant alleles of the cytochrome enzyme CYP2C9 have been associated with reduced warfarin metabolism and hence an increased risk of bleeding. However, the authors of a systematic review and meta-analysis on CYP2C9 and its relationship with warfarin administration have called for further evidence of the cost-effectiveness and clinical utility of routine testing, before recommending it.[21]

Based on the public consultation organised by the Royal Society, it is clear that a wide range of research needs to be undertaken to reassure the public, particularly in the field of pharmacogenetics research.[22] Box 7.1 summarises the range of current and future research.

Box 7.1 Pharmacogenetics: themes of current and future research

Sample storage
Regulation
Privacy and confidentiality
Racial group differences
Genetic stratification – differences based on genotype
Information transfer to health care professionals
Insurance issues

Genetics and free will

How much, it might be asked, are we the prisoners of our genomes? In every-day thoughts and actions, how much is unchangeable by virtue of genetic 'programming', and how much is the product of real free will?[23] This question is of relevance to those who might wish for or advise a change in behaviour – which, after all, is something that primary care clinicians are often doing as they work in the best interests of their patients.

Case study

G is a 40-year-old car dealer who drinks too much by his own admission. His alcohol consumption is generally around 60 units per week, and has been so for some time. His responses to the CAGE questionnaire are positive, and his work is suffering. Investigations have revealed a high Gamma Glutamyl Transferase (GGT) blood level. His father was an alcoholic who died of oesophageal varices.

This case differs from others that have been considered so far in that it involves the psychology and behaviour of the patient to a far greater extent. There is a hint of a genetic loading to G's problem drinking, in his family history,[24] but, most importantly, the solution to the impending health problem is in his own hands. No doubt clinicians will wish to support him in his efforts to curtail his drinking in whatever way is appropriate, but in the end the prognosis is self-determined.

Herein lies the genetic angle. Does G's family history mean that he is much less able to control his drinking by sheer effort of will? Alternatively, does it mean that G is fated to become an alcoholic because of his genetic loading? These questions of heritability are more difficult to answer in the area of behavioural genetics. We have seen that gene penetrance is variable in the context of physical disease – that is, the degree to which genotype is expressed into phenotype. It is immeasurably more difficult to assess genetic expression in the field of behaviour.[25]

Philosophers have one perspective on this issue, which they term *determinism*. A deterministic view of G would be that he is the prisoner of his genome, and that events could not turn out other than in his alcoholism. His free will is irrelevant or unavailable, and there is no role for his personal experiences in the modification of his fate. Nature will triumph over nurture. The term *genetic determinism* has been used to express this kind of view – that we are in fact the prisoners of our genes and cannot do other than that which they 'require' us to do. However, it is unlikely that this is so.

First, there is little empirical evidence that in the area of human behaviour, genes code for proteins which inevitably, and ultimately, determine actions.

Secondly, it makes little psychological sense that, given the wide range of possible contexts in which behaviours can occur, only one will actually happen. In the case of G, if this is so, whatever the life events he encounters, he will always be alcohol dependent.

Thirdly, it is important to acknowledge that there are situations in which genetic determinism is true. In the case of phenylketonuria,[26] those individuals who have the relevant genotype will turn out to have the phenotype as governed by the protein coding that follows. This analogy is not relevant to those less defined, polygenic traits that are involved in behaviours.

However, there is an interesting coda to this discussion of alcohol-related behaviour, and it is essentially monogenic and racial. The adverse effects of alcohol intoxication are associated with the breakdown product, acetaldehyde, which causes nausea, flushing and headache, among other things. The breakdown requires the alcohol dehydrogenase (ALDH) gene (or variants thereof) to code for the relevant enzymes. In South East Asia, the ALDH2*2 variant, which codes for a slow-metabolising form of the enzyme, is common, and the possession of this slow-ALDH allele seems to protect against alcoholism. This is a rare instance of a monogenic variation having a marked behavioural effect.

The wider issue of how behaviour might have a genetic basis has been explored in increasing depth in recent years. The details of this research are beyond the scope of this book, but some useful summary points should be made.

The more that connections are made between genotype and behaviour, the more danger there is of 'medicalising' behaviour, or characterising behaviours under various disease models. This has already happened in the case of alcoholism, and this has a clear empirical advantage, but it is less clear in other areas. The illusory nature of the 'gay gene'[27] substantiates this view. There is also the possibility that pre-implantation genetic diagnosis might be extended from its current application in serious disease, to traits such as intelligence or personality attributes. This is generally to be deplored.[28]

Future trends and developments

In the last section of this chapter, we shall take the liberty of indulging in some prognostication, perhaps even speculation, on the interaction between genetics and the primary care clinician in the years to come.

We consider that genetics will form more of the core work of primary care. There will be more conversations between clinicians and patients about what is 'bred in the bone.'[29] Some patients, informed by modern means of access to information, will seek to know more about their genetic risks, and how these may be moderated by environmental factors or behaviour. This inevitably will involve clinicians in complicated conversations, requiring relevant knowledge, about the interpretation of those risks. It will also require the traditional skills of good communication and *caritas*.[30] To this should be added, in view of the complexity of genetic knowledge, as revealed in this book, the skills of information searching and evaluation.

In this sense, the primary care clinician is not simply a traditional healer, but also an interface with the wider world of genetics – the more modern genetic knowledge that has become available in the last 20 years or so.

In 2007, the *British Medical Journal* offered the following list as summarising the key medical advances that have been made since 1840:[31]

1 anaesthesia
2 antibiotics
3 chlorpromazine
4 information technology
5 discovery of DNA
6 evidence-based medicine
7 microbiology
8 medical imaging
9 immunology
10 oral rehydration
11 oral contraception
12 knowing the risks of smoking
13 sanitation
14 tissue culture
15 vaccination.

Readers will no doubt have their own lists to offer, and as the *BMJ* notes, the list was initially informed by their readers' choices. Items 5 and 14 have clear genetic connections. Without tissue culture, we would not have *in-vitro* fertilisation, modern vaccines or karyotyping. Without DNA analysis, we would have no modern biology at all. It is a persuasive argument that this one advance holds the key to the future of medicine, which initially will be in the research environment, but will eventually trickle down to primary care. How might the primary care practitioner change his or her practice as a result in, say, 50 years' time?

It is our suspicion that patients will know much more about their individualised risks. The interrelationship between their genetic endowment and external risk factors should be better understood. Thus, as well as assessing patients' coronary artery disease risk simply in terms of lipids, smoking and the other risk factors considered in Chapter 4, clinicians will have more precise details about the overall risk. It will be personalised in the sense that where there is a family history, the genetic analysis of that risk should be more complete. The genes that code for the risk will be better understood, and their presence or absence in individuals will be known. Thus the internal risks of genetic loading can be evaluated with the external risks of, for example, smoking or alcohol.

Of itself, that individual knowledge might be considered valuable, but it may also cause patients to think, perhaps in a more fatalistic way, about their own lifespan. Already an issue for patients with monogenic disorders, it will thus become an issue for those with polygenic factors, too.

There are a number of research-level issues that are discussed in the public domain, but which are as yet of limited relevance to the primary care practitioner. Nonetheless, awareness of their future application may be useful in terms of general interest.

Cloning

Clones are genetically identical human beings, or indeed genetically identical animals or plants. Identical twins, for example, are naturally occurring clones. Cloning has been brought about already in lower animals, and famously in sheep. No human clones have been reported or confirmed yet. To clone a person would inevitably have enormous ethical implications, but technically it may become possible fairly soon. The clinical implications are hard to see, and cloning in humans is generally represented as the whim of strange, rich people who wish to reinvent themselves.

Stem-cell therapy

Stem cells are pluripotent cells that are found in early development. As they are capable of developing into virtually any kind of cell, they have the opportunity to be used as a source of replacement cells for diseased or abnormal cells. They can be sourced from human embryonic tissue or cadaveric fetal tissue, and therein lies the ethical difficulty. Those who would object to the use of this kind of tissue from embryo research or abortuses would resist research in the field.[32] Nonetheless, research is ongoing, and treatments are beginning to be offered in some areas (e.g. after bone-marrow ablation in leukaemia). Future therapies may be developed for severe neurological disease, including Parkinson's disease.

Germ-line manipulation

The term 'genetic engineering' loosely describes situations where the genome is manipulated, by insertion or deletion of DNA segments. If such a process is performed on differentiated cells, it is referred to as somatic cell manipulation. If it is performed on sperm or eggs before fertilisation, it is termed germ-line manipulation. Clearly in the latter case the change will be passed on to future generations. The procedure is not yet performed in humans, but if it was, it could have the capacity to alter 'adverse' genes and eradicate congenital disease. Germ-line manipulation is also fraught with ethical complications.

Chimaeras and hybrids

Chimaeras are entities that possess genetic material from two separate individuals. Thus body tissues are endowed with two separate genetic complements, usually as a result of embryo fusion. Hybrids are formed similarly, but are simply the result of genetic combination. The area is of importance in the research field because this kind of technology might be useful for redressing a shortage of stem-cell lines. At the time of writing, the UK Government is consulting on redrafting the law to include reference to these processes, as the hybridising of human and animal genes in research obviously has enormous implications. So far, the legislative drive is to allow hybrids for research, but to prohibit implantation in a woman.[33]

A new Lamarckism?

The final future trend we shall describe here is a fascinating recent finding from a European research team, who have observed that acquired change to humans may indeed cross the generations.[34] In their study populations, those boys who started smoking early were found to have sons with a higher body mass index (BMI). Furthermore, grandparental nutrition seemed to affect the mortality of grandsons. They concluded that these environmental factors have an effect that is trans-generational, and may reflect the classic Lamarckian inheritance of acquired change, no longer part of Darwinian biology. Clearly further research is required, but if this is a true finding, it may have implications for the advice that primary care clinicians can give their patients, as the impact on future generations suddenly becomes pertinent.

After this diversion into higher research, let us return to the theme mentioned at the beginning of this section. The traditional skills of primary care are based on caring for individuals, and will be more useful than ever in the age of genetic medicine. Although health care professionals might become more knowledgeable and skilled in the genetic area (and we hope that they do), it is their traditional skills which will be the building blocks for working in the 'genetically literate' age.

There are likely to be many challenges ahead for primary care. These will range from genetic risk assessment, and the diagnosis and understanding of the clinical utility of genetic testing, through to the coordination of care of people with genetic conditions. The challenges will include dealing with the ethical dilemmas that might be faced by individual patients, their families or society as a whole.

The important principle is that there is a basic understanding of the potential impact of clinical genetics within primary care. As Dr Frances Collins of the US National Human Genome Research Institute has stated,[35] 'the foundation stone of the genomic era, the Human Genome Project, has been laid.' Collins and colleagues suggest that the translation from genomics to biology, health and society will lead to scientific advances through the resources, technology development and the power of computational biology. However, if healthcare professionals are to rise to this new world of genomic medicine, they will need to be trained, educated and able to deal with the ethical, legal and social issues and dilemmas that will undoubtedly arise.

References

1. Nelkin D, Andrews L. DNA identification and surveillance creep. In: Conrad P, Gabe J, editors. *Social Perspectives on the New Genetics.* Oxford: Blackwell Publishers; 1999. This chapter deals with the larger questions about DNA testing, mainly from the American perspective.

2. www.parliament.uk/documents/upload/postpn258.pdf (accessed 2 January 2007).

3. For a discussion of this aspect, as well as most other areas of general genetic interest, see www.genewatch.org

4. The prevailing moral climate seems to support a child's right to know their biological parentage. If this is true, it is not the same thing as a parental right to know.

5. Human Genetics Commission. *Genes Direct: ensuring the oversight of genetic tests supplied directly to the public.* London: Human Genetics Commission; 2003. p. 23; www.hgc.gov.uk/UploadDocs/DocPub/Document/genesdirect_full.pdf

6. Ibid.

7. Ibid.

8. Kumar S, Gantley M. Tensions between policy makers and general practitioners in implementing the new genetics. *BMJ.* 1999; **319:** 140–3.

9. McCunney RJ. Genetic testing: ethical implications in the workplace. *Occup Med.* 2002; **17:** 665–72.

10. For US Congress details, see http://olpa.od.nih.gov/tracking/109/house_bills/session1/hr-1227.asp (accessed 1 March 2007).

11. For full text, see www.opsi.gov.uk/acts/acts1995/1995050.htm (accessed 1 March 2007).

12. Human Genetics Commission. *Inside Information: balancing interests in the use of personal genetic data.* London: Human Genetics Commission; 2002.

13. Hansard. House of Lords debate. *Genetic Testing: employment and insurance,* 15 March 2006.

14. McNally R. *Post-eugenics, 'eubionics' and the 'handicap ground' for abortion;* http://genome.wellcome.ac.uk/doc%5Fwtd020978.html (accessed 2 February 2007).

15. Lederberg J. Molecular biology, eugenics and euphenics. *Nature.* 1963; **198:** 428–9.

16. Moore P. *Babel's Shadow.* London: Lion; 2000. A very readable science journalist's perspective on all aspects of modern genetics.

17. Roses A. Pharmacogenetics' place in modern medical science and practice. *Life Sci.* 2002; **70:** 1471–80.

18. www.wellcome.ac.uk/doc_WTD003500.html 2.12.06.

19. Nuffield Council on Bioethics. *Pharmacogenetics: ethical issues.* London: Nuffield Council on Bioethics; 2002.

20. Royal Society. *Personalised Medicines: hopes and realities.* London: Royal Society; 2005.

21. Sanderson S, Emery J, Higgins J. CYP2CP gene variants, drug dose and bleeding risk in warfarin-treated patients: a HuGEnet systematic review and meta-analysis. *Genet Med.* 2005; **7:** 97–104.

22. Royal Society. *Pharmacogenetics Dialogue.* London: Royal Society; 2005.

23. Greenspan PS. Free will and the genome project. In: Nelson JL, Nelson HL, editors. *Meaning and Medicine: a reader in the philosophy of health care.* London: Routledge; 1999. A very engaging series of essays on various medico-philosophical subjects.

24. Cooper B. Nature, nurture and mental disorder: old concepts in the new millennium. *Br J Psychiatry.* 2001; **178 (Suppl. 40):** S91–101. A comprehensive and accessible review of genetic influences on psychiatric disorder.

25. Song R. In: *Human Genetics: fabricating the future.* London: Darton, Longman and Todd; 2002. An interesting development and background to this area, with a Christian perspective, that may be of relevance to some readers.

26. In PKU, there is a recessive allele on chromosome 12 coding for phenylalanine hydroxylase.

27. Manson C. Presenting behavioural genetics: spin, ideology and our narrative interests. *J Med Ethics.* 2004: **30:** 601–4. A review of the Nuffield Council's report on behavioural genetics,28 with reference to the distortions of publicity about behavioural genetics.

28. Nuffield Council on Bioethics. *Genetics and Human Behaviour: the ethical context.* London: Nuffield Council on Bioethics; 2002. A full examination of the area of behavioural genetics.

29. An old saying, but also the title of one component of *The Cornish Trilogy,* a wonderful series of books by the Canadian author Robertson Davies, who had much to say about doctors. Penguin; 1991, ISBN 0140144463.

30. *Caritas,* part of the motto of the Royal College of General Practitioners in the UK, denotes the quality of caring for the patient.

31. *Medical Milestones. BMJ.* 2007; **334 (Suppl. 1)**.

32. Singer P. Creating embryos. In: Mappes TA, DeGrazia D, editors. *Biomedical Ethics.* 4th ed. McGraw-Hill; 1996, ISBN 0-07-040141-1.

33. For a summary of current recommendations, see www.dh.gov.uk/PolicyAndGuidance/HealthAndSocialCareTopics/StemCell/StemCellGeneralInformation/StemCellGeneralArticle/fs/en?CONTENT_ID=4124082&chk=5mbZjS. 2.12.06.

34. Pembrey M, Bygren LO *et al.* Sex-specific, male-line transgenerational responses in humans. *Eur J Hum Genet.* 2006; **14:** 159–66.

35. Collins FS *et al.* A vision for the future of genomics research. *Nature.* 2003; **422:** 1–13.

8

Resources for the primary health care professional

Introduction

This chapter will tease out useful sources of further information about primary care genetics from among the myriad resources currently available. It will highlight some of the sources, both paper and electronic, already referred to that are most useful to the general primary care reader. References already cited in the text are chosen where they amplify meaning, rather than merely as an academic or bureaucratic process. Sources that are directly useful to patients are also included. The whole area was well reviewed in 2002, and interested readers are directed to this source in particular.[1] As a resource list, this chapter seeks to address the 'challenge of integrating genetic medicine into primary care.'[2]

Genetic 'interest' groups

This section will identify and describe some of the most useful sources of information for the primary care professional, both as part of day-to-day work and for the more interested reader. It has been a theme of this book that the genetic care field is moving into primary care, and also that this is a good thing. Inevitably, this has consequences for the personal development of clinicians, which we shall address.

Those working in the UK will usually be part of the National Health Service (as there is very little primary care outwith the NHS), and are therefore able to access specialist genetic care relatively easily. That may or may not be the case in other countries, and the international angle is dealt with below.

Electronic resources are deliberately given priority. This is not to deny the value of the printed word (indeed many books have been referenced thus far), but simply to highlight the variety of methods of learning that are available on the Internet.

The National Genetics and Education Centre

www.geneticseducation.nhs.uk
The aims and objectives of this organisation have been described in chapter 2. Two areas within the site are of particular interest to practising clinicians who may not be 'genetically aware.'

The 'Learning Genetics' section contains sources divided by profession, and subsections on the following:

- understanding genetics
- patterns of inheritance
- family history
- genetic testing and screening
- ethical, legal and social implications of genetics
- communicating genetic information.

The 'Genetics in Practice' section contains summary descriptions of most of the major genetic diseases (other than multifactorial ones), and advice on drawing a family tree.

www.geneticseducation.nhs.uk/learning/learning_genetics.asp
www.geneticseducation.nhs.uk/practice/index.asp?id=4

For those of a more academic disposition, there is a full reading list of articles about primary care genetics:

www.geneticseducation.nhs.uk/publications/primary_care.asp

The Human Genetics Commission (HGC)

www.hgc.gov.uk/Client/index.asp?ContentId=1

This body advises the UK Government on genetics and genetic policy. It is primarily concerned with social and ethical issues. As a public and open organisation, its membership is wide but its influence is considerable. Readers who are seeking more general content as a background to their clinical care will find much of interest here.

The HGC maintains interest groups for the following areas:

- identity testing
- genetic services
- intellectual property aspects
- genetic databases
- genetic decision making in reproduction
- genetic discrimination
- genetic profiles of new babies.

More than anything else, the site outlines the HGC opinion as offered to the public and UK law makers.

PEGASUS (Professional Education for Genetic Assessment and Screening)

www.pegasus.nhs.uk

Already referred to in Chapter 2, this organisation promotes the development of special skills in genetics for all health care professionals, and trains the future genetics trainers. There is a focus on haemoglobinopathies, but all aspects of genetic screening are covered.

The Genetics Interest Group (GIG)

www.gig.org.uk/index.html

This is primarily an umbrella organisation that promotes awareness and understanding of genetic conditions. However, its website contains a wealth of useful material for the clinician, including:

- an index of regional genetics centres (www.gig.org.uk/services.htm)
- some good basic genetics (www.gig.org.uk/education2.htm)
- some interesting videos about living with genetic conditions, that will also be useful and informative for health care professionals (www.gig.org.uk/clips.htm).

GIG also provides information for many Government consultations, and seeks to maximise genetic services.

Royal College of General Practitioners (RCGP)

www.rcgp.org.uk/PDF/curr 6 Genetics in Primary Care.pdf
Having recently produced a full curriculum for GP training, the RCGP now has a formal content list for genetics. This defines the core knowledge and skills relevant to clinical general practice in the UK, and it is relevant to primary care anywhere in the developed world. At the time of writing, this curriculum is being implemented for the new generation of GP trainees, but it will have implications for all.

British Society for Human Genetics

www.bshg.org.uk
This is the primary organisation that represents the views of genetics professionals in the UK. There are interesting policy documents that are worth examining and relevant to primary care, as well as links to affiliated groups such as the Association of Genetic Nurses and Counsellors.

The Public Health Genetics Unit in Cambridge

www.phgu.org.uk
This is an excellent resource, relevant to primary care, particularly looking at the ethical, legal and social consequences of clinical genetics. It keeps abreast of service implications and public health policy.

OMNI (Organising Medical Networked Information)

http://omni.ac.uk
This is essentially a gateway to biomedical Internet resources organised through the University of Nottingham.

Primary Care Genetics Society

http://pcgs.org.uk
This is a newly formed society that will aim to raise awareness of genetic medicine in primary care.

Genomics Policy Research Unit, University of Glamorgan

http://genomics.research.glam.ac.uk/community/rss
This functions to develop the impact of genetics, and has a multidisciplinary perspective.

Ethox: Oxford Genetics and Society Research Programme

www.ethox.org.uk/research/genetics/parker.htm

This focuses on the ethical, legal and societal impact of genetics and has a link to GenEthics (www.ethox.org.uk/Genethics/index.htm), a special interest group of the British Society for Human Genetics, which looks at ethical dilemmas in genetics.

Patient support groups

Most individual genetic disease is fairly rare and specialised, although the totality of genetic disease is not. Therefore support groups, as well as being of interest to patients, may well be useful to clinicians as a means of helping them to care for individuals with genetic disease. Websites appropriate to them are listed alphabetically below. The authors do not necessarily endorse their content, but have found them to be useful in clinical or academic practice.

Adrenoleucodystrophy

www.aldfst.org.uk
A family support site, orientated towards children.

Alkaptonuria

www.alkaptonuria.info/home.html
Multilingual site with much clinical information and good links. Recommended.

Alport syndrome

www.rarediseases.org/search/rdbdetail_abstract.html?disname=Alport%20Syndrome
US site with good links to all renal disease information.

Alström syndrome

www.alstrom.org.uk/default.asp
Includes a good section for clinicians.

Angelman syndrome

www.angelmanuk.org
Minimal clinical information, but useful for families.

Aniridia

www.geocities.com/aniridia_uk
Primarily a support group network.

Anorchidism

http://freespace.virgin.net/asg.uk
Contains brief clinical details and patients' stories.

Ataxia-telangiectasia

www.atsociety.org.uk
Mainly a fundraising site.

Batten's disease

www.bdfa-uk.org.uk/index.htm
Contains useful clinical summaries, but light on detail.

Beckwith–Weideman syndrome

www.bws-support.org.uk
Contains excellent technical genetic information.

Charcot–Marie–Tooth disease

www.cmt.org.uk/index.php?option=com_content&task=view&id=77&Itemid=100
Full of specialist information that will be helpful to clinicians.

Cornelia de Lange syndrome

www.cdls.org.uk/information/12.htm
Beautifully laid out sections, and strong on clinical content.

Costello syndrome

www.costellokids.co.uk/welcome.htm
Unusually full site, with patients' stories and videos, as well as clinical content.

Cri du chat syndrome

www.criduchat.co.uk
Much useful clinical content.

Cystic fibrosis

www.cftrust.org.uk
Offers a good patient forum facility.

DiGeorge syndrome

www.maxappeal.org.uk
Explains the condition in terms of the symptoms.

Ectodermal dysplasia

www.ectodermaldysplasia.org/frame.htm
Mainly for families, but with links to many scientific papers.

Edward's syndrome

www.soft.org.uk
Family support for trisomy 18 and other trisomies.

Ehlers–Danlos syndrome

www.ehlers-danlos.org/eds.htm
Full clinical information in a well-designed site.

Epidermolysis bullosa

www.debra.org.uk/research
Good coverage of professional information and family support.

Familial adenomatous polyposis

www.fapgene.org.uk/index.html
Consists mainly of powerful patients' stories.

Fragile X syndrome

www.fragilex.org.uk
Contains very useful contributions from leaders in the field.

Gaucher's disease

www.gaucher.org.uk/contents.htm
Blend of research information and patient support (English, Spanish and Russian versions available).

Gilbert's syndrome

www.gilbertssyndrome.org.uk
Brief site with some unsubstantiated advice for patients.

Gorlin's syndrome

www.gorlingroup.co.uk/index.htm
Full information for families and clinicians.

Haemochromatosis

www.gorlingroup.co.uk/index.htm
Very accessible site for families and clinicians.

Haemophilia, Von Willebrand's disease and other bleeding disorders

www.haemophilia.org.uk/index.php
Well-designed site, but low on detail for clinicians.

Homocystinuria

www.hcusupport.com
Quite simple support site by a US patient.

Huntington's disease

www.hda.org.uk
Excellent fact sheets to download.

Ito's disease

www.e-fervour.com/hits/#hits
Mainly for family support.

Jervell and Lange-Nielsen syndrome

www.rarediseases.org/search/rdbdetail_abstract.html?disname=Jervell%20and%20Lange-Nielsen%20Syndrome
Brief US review.

Klinefelter syndrome

www.klinefelter.org.uk/Main1.html
Useful clinical information for clinicians and for affected boys and their parents.

Lawrence–Moon–Bardet–Biedl syndrome

www.lmbbs.org.uk/about.htm
Helpful information, mainly for families.

Lowe syndrome

www.lowetrust.com/index.html
Excellent links to other relevant sites.

Marfan's syndrome

http://marfan.org.uk/component/option,combfrontpage/Itemid,1
Slightly untidy site, with only basic information.

Mowat–Wilson syndrome

www.mowatwilsonsyndrome.co.uk
Only contains basic medical information, but has good links to other sites.

Muscular dystrophy

www.muscular-dystrophy.org/index.html
Excellent fact sheets in a campaigning site.

Neurofibromatosis

www.nfauk.org
Very comprehensive site.

Osteopetrosis

www.osteopetrosis.co.uk
Mainly consists of carers' stories.

Patau's syndrome

www.soft.org.uk
Family support for trisomy 13 and other trisomies.

Pendred's syndrome

www.madisonsfoundation.org/content/3/1/display.asp?did=560
Highly informative US site for families.

Phenylketonuria

www.nspku.org
Useful basic information for parents and clinicians.

Porphyria

www.porphyria.org.uk/facts.htm
Easily understood classification of types, but at a superficial level.

Prader–Willi syndrome

www.ppuk.org/site.php?action=page&pageID=1
Good information for families, but less useful for professionals.

Pseudoxanthoma elasticum

www.pxe.org.uk/pages/aboutpixie.html
Mainly family-orientated content.

Retinitis pigmentosa

www.brps.org.uk
Very patient-friendly site, and also useful for clinicians.

Rett syndrome

www.rettsyndrome.org.uk
Brief clinical descriptions, mainly family-orientated content.

Rubinstein–Taybi syndrome

www.rtsuk.org/home/index.asp
Includes a good patient forum facility.

Shwachman–Diamond syndrome

www.shwachman-diamondsupport.org
Includes a good patient forum facility.

Sickle-cell disease

www.sicklecellsociety.org
Includes a good patient forum facility.

Stickler syndrome

www.stickler.org.uk
Very impressive content, arranged for professionals and families separately.

Thalassaemia

www.ukts.org
Very comprehensive site.

Treacher–Collins syndrome

www.treachercollins.net/syndrome.html
Useful for clinicians and families, and very well laid out.

Tuberous sclerosis

www.tuberous-sclerosis.org
Excellent content on research, with expert commentaries.

Turner's syndrome

www.tss.org.uk/whatis.htm
Full of information both for clinicians and for women with this diagnosis.

Usher syndrome

www.sense.org.uk/deafblindness/usher
Fine site from the British group *SENSE* for all deaf/blind patients.

Waardenburg's syndrome

www.mamashealth.com/ear/waar.asp
Contains brief information for relatives.

Wolf–Hirshhorn syndrome

www.whs.webk.co.uk
Explanatory information, but at a simple level.

Worster-Drought syndrome (congenital suprabulbar paresis)

www.wdssg.org.uk/whatiswds.php
Mainly a discussion forum, with good links to some relevant research papers.

Xeroderma pigmentosum

www.xpsupportgroup.org.uk
Patient-orientated site with many newsletters to members, but little clinical
detail.

X-linked hypophosphataemia (vitamin D-resistant rickets)

www.xlhnetwork.org
Good clinical detail.

European and worldwide resources

Genetics as a subject obviously knows no national boundaries, and therefore
there is an enormous body of literature in the public domain from around the
world. For UK readers, that perspective can be gained by visiting any of the
sources of information in other countries. The authors find the following
resources most useful in clinical and education practice.

Centre for Genetics Education (Australia)

www.genetics.com.au/conditions/default.htm
This site offers excellent information on monogenic disorders as summaries for
clinicians, a glossary of terms and downloadable fact sheets.

US Department of Health and Human Sciences: Centres for Disease Control and Prevention

www.cdc.gov

Under this website is a link to the centres and the genomics centre. One of its key resources is the Human Genome Epidemiology Network (HuGENet), which is a rich vein of reviews, collaborative work and resources for anyone who is particularly interested in the public health aspects of genomics.

National Coalition for Health Professionals in Education in Genetics

www.nchpeg.org

This US organisation is the equivalent of the National Genetics Education Centre – a collaboration of many organisations whose remit is to help to develop genetics education.

Bioethical resources from around the world

A good links summary of the contributions of individual countries to this field is to be found on the UK Human Genetics Commission website at www.hgc.gov.uk/Client/Content_wide.asp?ContentId=144

Genetics Tools Home Page (University of Washington, USA)

www.genetests.org/servlet/access?id=8888892&key=HaqLJxUABDXXp&fcn=y&f w=Luva&filename=/tools/index.html

This unwieldy URL conceals a wealth of teaching and learning material, subtitled 'Genetics with a Primary Care Lens.' Cases have been worked up from primary care, with analysis in biological and social terms.

National Coalition of Health Professional Education in Genetics (NCHPEG)

www.nchpeg.org

This US site contains a wealth of material for all health care professionals, not only clinicians. It is available in English and Spanish. Slide shows of the last few years' meetings cover virtually all subjects of interest to those in primary care.

References

1. Emery J, Burke W. Genetics education for primary care providers. *Nature.* 2002; **3:** 561–6.

2. Emery J, Hayflick S. The challenge of integrating genetic medicine into primary care. *BMJ.* 2001; **322:** 1027–30.

Further reading

This section draws together books that have been referenced in the preceding chapters, and adds more. Again the criterion for inclusion in this list is simply

that the authors have found them useful and informative, and an aid to understanding. Journal papers mentioned previously are not listed here.

General reading about genetics

- Marantz Henig R. *A Monk and Two Peas: the story of Gregor Mendel and the discov-
  ery of genetics.* London: Wiedenfeld and Nicolson; 2000.
- Gould SJ. *Dinosaur in a Haystack: reflections in natural history.* London: Jonathan
  Cape; 1996.
- Moore P. *Babel's Shadow.* London: Lion; 2000.
- Harris J. *Clones, Genes and Immortality: ethics and the genetics revolution.* Oxford:
  Oxford University Press; 1998.
- Song R. *Human Genetics: fabricating the future.* London: Darton, Longman and
  Todd; 2002.
- Petersen A, Bunton R. *The New Genetics and the Public's Health.* London:
  Routledge; 2002.
- Duster T. *Backdoor to Eugenics.* London: Routledge; 1990.

Clinical genetics

- Lindee S. *Moments of Truth in Genetic Medicine.* Baltimore, MD: Johns Hopkins
  University Press; 2005.
- Clarke A. *Genetic Counselling: practice and principles.* London: Routledge; 1994.
- Harper PS. Genetic counselling: an introduction. In: *Practical Genetic
  Counselling.* Oxford: Butterworth-Heinemann; 2000.

Genetics and ethics

- Nuffield Council on Bioethics. *Genetics and Human Behaviour: the ethical context.*
  London: Nuffield Council on Bioethics; 2002.
- Joint Committee on Medical Genetics. *Consent and Confidentiality in Genetic
  Practice: guidance on genetic testing and sharing genetic information.* London: Royal
  College of Physicians, Royal College of Pathologists and British Society for
  Human Genetics; 2006.
- Beauchamp TL, Childress JF. *Principles of Biomedical Ethics.* 4th ed. Oxford:
  Oxford University Press; 2001.
- Rachels J. *Elements of Moral Philosophy.* 2nd ed. McGraw-Hill; 1995.
- Dworkin R. *Life's Dominion: an argument about abortion, euthanasia and individ-
  ual freedom.* London: Vintage Press; 1994.
- Harris J, editor. *Bioethics.* Oxford: Oxford University Press; 2001.
- Mappes TA, DeGrazia D, editors. *Biomedical Ethics.* 4th ed. McGraw-Hill; 1996.
- Nelson JL, Nelson HL, editors. *Meaning and Medicine: a reader in the philosophy
  of health care.* London: Routledge; 1999.
- Conrad P, Gabe J, editors. *Social Perspectives on the New Genetics.* Oxford:
  Blackwell Publishers; 1999.

Genetics and reproduction

- Louhiala P. *Preventing Intellectual Disability*. Cambridge: Cambridge University Press; 2004.
- Heyd D. *Genethics: moral issues in the creation of people*. Berkeley, CA: University of California Press; 1994.

Glossary of terms

Acrocentric Having the centromere located near one end of the chromosome.

Allele Alternative forms of a gene that are responsible for alternative traits.

Altruism The situation in which one person benefits another without there necessarily being a pay-off.

Aneuploidy The presence of more or fewer than the usual (diploid) number of chromosomes, giving rise to an abnormal chromosome number. There may be partial aneuploidy, where there is the addition or loss of part of a chromosome.

Anticipation Through successive generations a worsening of the severity of a disease, which may occur at a younger age.

Autonomy literally 'self-rule' – the ability of an individual to decide their own future.

Autosome One of 22 pairs of chromosomes other than the X or Y chromosome.

Base pair A pair of complementary nitrogenous bases that bond to form 'rungs' on the DNA double helix. Adenine (A) bonds with thymine (T), and cytosine (C) bonds with guanine (G).

Candidate gene A gene suspected of causing disease and located in a chromosomal region under study.

Centromere The region of the chromosome where spindle attachment occurs during cell division.

Chimaera An organism consisting of two or more cells originating from different zygotes.

Chromatin Material consisting of DNA (in a condensed state) and associated proteins.

Clinical utility The value or usefulness of a test for distinguishing between disease and normality.

Clinical validity The usefulness of a test for distinguishing between an affected and an unaffected individual. It takes into account the sensitivity, specificity and predictive value of the test used.

Cloning The generation of genetically identical cells or organisms from a single ancestral origin.

Consanguinity A relationship between blood relatives with a common ancestor. In this context it refers mainly to marriages between cousins.

Consequentialism Moral theory that defines the right actions by their consequences.

Consultand The person who is seeking genetic advice about a genetic disorder.

Deletion The loss of part of a DNA sequence or part of a chromosome.

De novo Arising from new rather than being inherited.

Determinism A philosophical term describing the situation where there is only one possible outcome of events, which cannot be altered.

Dizygotic twins Two individuals produced from two separate eggs that were fertilised by two separate sperm.

DNA (deoxyribonucleic acid) The genetic information of living organisms. It has a double-stranded helical molecule, and is found in the nucleus of cells. The two strands of the helix are bound together by bonds between pairs of nucleotides (base pairs).

Dominant Describing a mutant allele which may lead to disease despite the presence of the normal allele.

Eubionics The quest for bodily perfection.

Eugenics The use and manipulation of selective breeding to improve the genotype of future generations.

Euphenics The improvement of phenotype.

Exon A segment of a gene that codes for the synthesis of a protein.

Expressivity The variability in the severity of a genetic disorder.

Familial adenomatous polyposis coli (FAP) An autosomal dominant condition that gives rise to colonic polyposis and is associated with a high risk of developing cancer of the colon.

Fluorescence *in situ* hybridisation (FISH) The labelling of a DNA probe with a fluorescent tag which then binds to a specific chromosomal region. This can be visualised by fluorescence microscopy.

Frameshift mutation An alteration of the reading frame of the gene, due to either deletion or insertion that is not a multiple of three base pairs.

Gamete A male sperm cell or female egg cell.

Gene A sequence of DNA that encodes a protein or RNA. It is the basic unit of heredity.

Genetics counselling The giving of advice to patients or families about the possibility of developing the genetic disorder under discussion through inheritance.

Genome All of the genetic material that is contained within chromosomes.

Genotype The genetic make-up that characterises the physical traits, contained within functioning cells.

Germ cells The cells that give rise to sperm cells or egg cells.

Haploid Having a set of autosomal chromosomes and one sex chromosome (i.e. 23, X or 23, Y), as occurs in gametes.

Haplotype A set of closely linked alleles on a chromosome.

Hemizygous Having only one copy of a gene.

Hereditary Relating to the genetic transfer of information from parent to offspring.

Hereditary non-polyposis coli (HNPCC) A dominantly inherited condition that causes polyps in the colon, with an inherited tendency to develop cancer.

Heterozygous Having different alleles on the same locus on a chromosome.

Histone protein The protein structure around which DNA is coiled.

Homozygous Having two identical alleles on the same locus.

Human leucocyte antigen (HLA) The HLA system codes for antigens present on cell surfaces.

Inherited Genetic information that is passed on from parent to offspring, giving rise to a trait or condition from the parent.

Intron A non-coding segment of DNA, located in between the coding exons.

***In-vitro* fertilisation (IVF)** Fertilisation of a woman's eggs with sperm outside the uterus, followed by transfer of the embryo into the uterus.

Karyotype The chromosomal characteristics of a cell or of an individual.

Locus The position of a gene on a chromosome.

Meiosis The division of diploid cells to form haploid cells or gametes.

Microsatellite instability Microsatellites are short stretches of DNA which are repeated. During mitosis there may be varying lengths of microsatellites.

Missense mutation An altered amino acid due to a nucleotide substitution.

Mitosis Cell division that results in two equal daughter cells with identical sets of chromosomes.

Monosomy One copy of a chromosome.

Monozygotic twins A single fertilised egg that separates into two identical embryos and individuals.

Moral relativism The philosophical situation in which morality is defined by groups rather than universally.

Mosaicism Two or more cell populations.

Multifactorial disease Disease that results from an interaction between genes and the environment.

Mutation A permanent change in the genetic material. This leads to a change in the function of the gene product, and it is transmissible to the offspring.

Non-disjunction During meiosis, failure of chromosome pairs to separate into daughter cells.

Nucleotide One purine or pyrimidine base combined with an attached phosphate group and sugar molecule.

Penetrance The probability that a disease genotype will show an abnormal phenotype.

Phenotype The outward and physical appearance of an individual.

Polymerase chain reaction (PCR) The amplification and replication of DNA sequences through a process that involves denaturing DNA.

Polymorphisms The natural variations in DNA sequence between different members of a population, or within a species.

Predictive Trying to project for the future.

Premutation A mutation that will probably lead to an abnormal phenotypic effect in subsequent generations. Most carriers of a premutation are unaffected.

Prevalence The proportion of people who are affected by a particular disease at a given time.

Proband The index case through which the family history is ascertained.

Protein A large molecule, necessary for growth and development, which is composed of amino acids linked by peptide bonds.

Recessive Relating to a genetic trait or disease that is only manifested when both alleles are altered.

Rights A moral theory in which social relationships between individuals imply obligations and duties.

Sensitivity The ability of a test to detect a disease or a condition when it is present.

Sequencing The determination of the genetic code in DNA or RNA. It involves elucidation of the order of the nucleotides.

Specificity The proportion of people who are free of a particular disease who have a negative test.

Telomere Either of the two tips of a chromosome.

Transgenic Referring to modification of the genome of an organism by the introduction of new DNA into the germ line.

Trisomy Three copies of a chromosome.

Utilitarianism Moral theory describing the greatest good for the greatest number.

Value The worth, quality or utility of something.

Virtue Moral theory according to which the personal attributes of the agent are the descriptor, rather than the action under consideration.

X-linked inheritance A trait or disease that is due to the presence of altered genes on the X chromosome.

Zygote A fertilised ovum.

Index